What You Really Need to Know about Moles and Melanoma

A

JOHNS

HOPKINS

PRESS

HEALTH BOOK

WHAT YOU REALLY

NEED TO KNOW

ABOUT MOLES

AND MELANOMA

. . .

Jill R. Schofield, M.D., and
William A. Robinson, M.D., Ph.D.

THE JOHNS HOPKINS UNIVERSITY PRESS
Baltimore & London

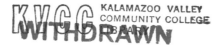

Note to the reader: This book is not meant to substitute for medical care of people with melanoma, and treatment should not be based solely on its contents. Instead, treatment must be developed in a dialogue between the individual and his or her physician. Our book has been written to help with that dialogue.

© 2000 The Johns Hopkins University Press
All rights reserved. Published 2000
Printed in the United States of America on acid-free paper
9 8 7 6 5 4 3 2 1

The Johns Hopkins University Press
2715 North Charles Street
Baltimore, Maryland 21218-4363
www.press.jhu.edu

Library of Congress Cataloging-in-Publication Data will be found at the end of this book.

A catalog record for this book is available from the British Library.
ISBN 0-8018-6393-7
ISBN 0-8018-6394-5 (pbk.)

Illustrations on pages 5, 7, 10, 17, 24, 26, 28, 67, 86, and 107 by Jacqueline Schaffer.

Illustrations on pages 1, 75, and 147 courtesy the Anti-Cancer Council of Victoria.

Dedicated to our patients—
past, present, and future

Contents

PART I. MELANOMA
Recognizing and Preventing It

PART II. MELANOMA
Diagnosis and Treatment

PART III. MELANOMA
Less Common Types and Melanoma Research

A gallery of color images follows page 36.

Preface

In Caucasians throughout the world, the incidence of malignant melanoma is increasing more rapidly than that of any other form of cancer. In recent years, medical literature has begun referring to melanoma as a modern epidemic. If the current rate of increase continues, by the early twenty-first century, the incidence of melanoma will probably be greater than the incidence of lung, colon, prostate, or breast cancer. This dramatic increase in melanoma is largely the result of increasingly intense sun exposure due to major changes in lifestyle and clothing styles in recent decades.

In most cases, melanoma is simply a form of skin cancer. In contrast to the more common skin cancers (**squamous cell** and **basal cell carcinomas**), however, melanoma has the potential of spreading to the rest of the body.[1] Furthermore, melanoma frequently occurs in young, otherwise healthy people in the prime of their lives. Fortunately, like cervical and colon cancers, melanoma has a known precursor, or **premalignant** stage, which can be identified in most cases by a simple skin examination. Removing the premalignant cells will prevent the potentially lethal cancerous cells from developing. In addition, there are known risk factors that allow us to identify people at highest risk for developing the disease.

Our ability to identify high-risk populations, avoid dangerous sun exposure, and remove premalignant lesions should make invasive melanoma a largely preventable disease. Unfortunately, the rapidity with which melanoma has become a major health problem has left both the public and health care professionals struggling to meet its

---

[1]Throughout this book, terms appearing in **boldface** are defined in the Glossary.

challenges. Public awareness of the dangers of melanoma and the importance of prevention and early detection needs to be improved. Physicians need to be better trained to pick up warning signs. More sensitive diagnostic tools need to be developed. And more effective treatments need to be found.

This book was written with the goal of helping people understand melanoma. We hope that it will help people avoid developing the disease. For people who already have melanoma and the families of these people, we hope it will help them understand what is happening to them and aid them in finding the best possible care.

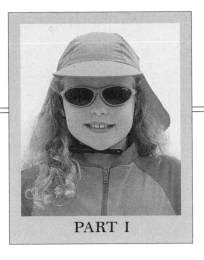

PART I

MELANOMA
Recognizing and Preventing It

Melanoma is largely a preventable disease
which is increasing in incidence because of
our modern lifestyle. Taking a variety of
factors into account, it is possible to
determine one's personal level of risk of
developing the disease. We can all reduce
this risk by minimizing exposure to the sun
and monitoring our moles for specific, well-
known warning signs.

What Is Malignant Melanoma?

*C*ancer is one of the most frightening words in the English language. Fortunately, by learning more about cancer, physicians and scientists have made great strides in preventing and treating this group of diseases. While these experts continue to look for better ways of preventing, diagnosing, and treating cancer, the nonscientific public is becoming better informed about how to avoid cancer-causing agents and how to look for and recognize symptoms that may indicate early stages of these diseases.

Some forms of cancer strike without warning, and we do not know why. With other kinds of cancer, we have learned a good deal about what causes them, and we have learned to spot their early warning signs. By acting on what we know about the causes and early signs of these cancers, we can go a long way toward protecting ourselves. Fortunately, melanoma falls in this second category. It is the purpose of this book to help people understand how and why melanoma develops and what steps they can take to avoid getting melanoma—or, if that is not possible, how to detect it early and get good treatment.

Malignant melanoma, usually referred to simply as **melanoma,** is a cancer that arises in the **melanocytes,** the cells that produce melanin. Most melanocytes are found in the skin, although they are also present in other parts of the body. **Melanin** is the pigment that gives our skin, hair, and eyes their color and that allows us to tan. Most melanomas (cancerous melanocytes) develop just below the skin's surface, usually at the site of an existing **mole.** If not removed promptly, melanoma cells can travel to all parts of the body and invade and destroy vital organs. This is what makes melanoma so dangerous.

Research has shown that the primary cause of melanoma is damage to the DNA of melanocytes by **ultraviolet** (UV) **radiation** from the sun (see Chapter 3). (**DNA,** or deoxyribonucleic acid, is the spiral-shaped structure in a cell that contains the genetic material that controls cell division and orchestrates all of the cell's "activities.") Our skin normally responds to sun exposure by making more melanin, and we see this increase in melanin as a tan. Melanin absorbs UV radiation and thereby protects our cells' DNA. When we are overexposed to the sun, however, and get too much UV radiation, the DNA may be damaged. People who produce more melanin, and darker melanin—generally darker-skinned people—are less likely to develop melanoma. Melanoma can occur in people of all skin types, however, and everyone should learn to recognize its danger signs.

THE STRUCTURE OF SKIN

We see our skin every day, but looking at it under a microscope is helpful in understanding how melanoma develops and how it is able to spread to the rest of the body. A drawing of the skin as it appears microscopically is shown in Figure 1.1.

The outermost layer of skin is called the **epidermis.** It is composed of cells called **keratinocytes.** The epidermis is very thin, on average only 1/25th of an inch thick. Nevertheless, it acts as a very effective barrier, protecting the body from bacteria and other microorganisms that are present everywhere in the environment but are too small to be seen with the naked eye.

The second layer of skin is called the *dermal layer,* or **dermis.** The dermis is much thicker than the epidermis and is composed primarily of fibers called *collagen,* which provide strength and structural support to the skin. (Leather is made from the dermal layer of cow skin.) The actual thickness of the dermis depends on its location; it is very thick on the back but is quite thin over the scalp or the top of the foot. The dermis is itself divided into two layers: the upper layer is called the *papillary dermis,* while the deeper layer is known as the *reticular dermis.* We will refer back to the two dermal layers when discussing the diagnosis of melanoma. The most important thing to know about the dermis is that, unlike the epidermis, it contains blood vessels and **lymphatic channels** (tiny vessels that carry the cells of

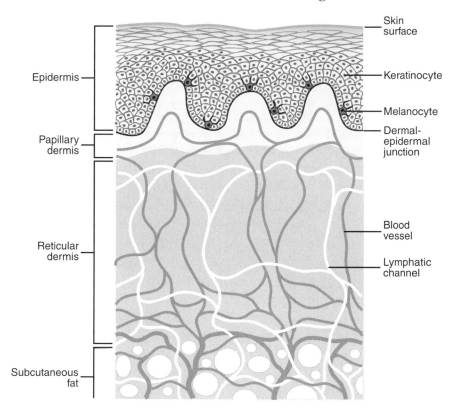

Epidermis

Papillary
dermis

Reticular
dermis

Subcutaneous
fat

Skin
surface

Keratinocyte

Melanocyte

Dermal-
epidermal
junction

Blood
vessel

Lymphatic
channel

FIGURE 1.1. The structure of skin: layers of the skin along with the blood supply and lymphatic channels. The top layer is the epidermis. Next comes the dermis, which has an upper layer (the papillary dermis) and a lower layer (the reticular dermis). Underneath these is a fat layer. The melanocytes are found along the junction where the epidermis and dermis join (the dermal-epidermal junction). Notice that the density of blood vessels and lymphatic channels increase in the deeper layers of skin, correlating with an increased risk of metastasis and melanoma recurrence with the most deeply invading lesions.

the immune system throughout the body). The number of blood vessels and lymphatic channels increases the deeper you go into the dermis (see Figure 1.1).

The third layer of the skin is called the **subcutaneous fat.** It is just that—fat. Its role is to allow us to maintain body heat. Fat, like the dermis, contains blood vessels and lymphatics, but more of them.

MELANOCYTES

Melanocytes are found in many places throughout the body—in the retina of the eye and in the linings of the mouth, nose, anus, rectum, vagina, and spinal cord. Most melanocytes, however, are found in the skin. The only known purpose of melanocytes is to make melanin to protect our skin cells from the sun's damaging UV rays. Scientists do not know what purpose these cells serve in non-skin locations, but it may be to detoxify potentially dangerous substances.

The melanocytes in the skin reside at the junction between the dermis and the epidermis (see Figure 1.1). On average, one in every ten cells found along the **dermal-epidermal junction** is a melanocyte; the others are keratinocytes. People with naturally dark skin do not have more melanocytes in their skin than lighter-skinned people. Rather, they make larger *amounts* of melanin, and they make a *darker form* of it. The melanin made inside the melanocytes is transferred along the cells' long arms (called *dendrites*) to neighboring keratinocytes in the epidermis. Melanoma arises when melanocyte cells begin to reproduce themselves in an uncontrolled fashion. When melanoma cells get into the blood vessels and lymphatic channels in the dermis, they can travel throughout the body.

WHAT IS CANCER?

To understand cancer, you have to understand how normal cells grow and function. All the normal cells in our body go through a normal cycle of growth, reproduction, and death. The process by which a cell produces another copy of itself is known as **cell division.** The process of repeated cell divisions is called **proliferation** (see Figure 1.2). Normally, cell division is a very carefully regulated process that ensures that the body has neither too few nor too many of a given cell type. Some cell types in the body are worn out quickly and need to be continuously replaced as they die. Examples include the cells that line the digestive tract and most of the blood cells. The proliferation of these cells must be precisely regulated based on their rate of cell death

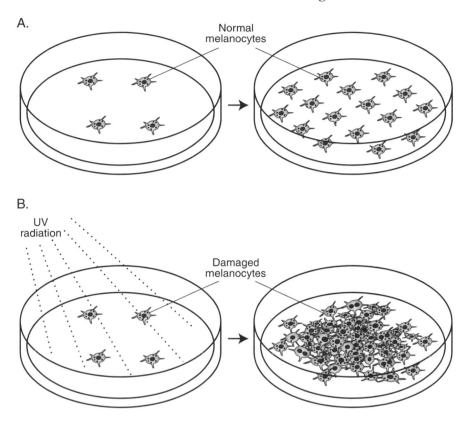

FIGURE 1.2. Cell proliferation: a comparison of how normal melanocytes and damaged melanocytes (melanoma cells) grow in the laboratory. Normal melanocytes (*A*) do not pile up on one another; they grow in a controlled way in the culture dish with space between the individual cells. The damaged melanocytes (*B*) pile on one another and grow in an uncontrolled way.

so that the body has the exact number of cells it needs; more or less would result in problems.

This regulation is achieved by signals generated in the "brain" of the cell, called the **nucleus,** and sent from cell to cell. The nucleus contains the cell's DNA, which in turn is composed of thousands of **genes.** Genes are simply stretches of precise DNA sequences. Each gene serves as a code or blueprint that instructs the body to produce a specific **protein.** Most people think of proteins as a type of food energy that helps build strong muscles. More technically, however, *protein* is the term for essential molecules in the body. The proteins are the "workhorses" of the cell.

Some proteins, such as the collagen in our skin, are important for the structure of muscles, tissues, and organs. Some have unique and critical jobs; insulin, for example, is a protein that regulates our blood sugar level. Other proteins, including some hormones, are involved in directing a cell to become a skin cell or a brain cell or a liver cell. Still other proteins are crucial in regulating the speed at which a specific cell type can proliferate. It is these growth regulatory proteins that are vitally important in controlling cell proliferation. Genes are equally important because any error (**mutation**) in the DNA sequence (gene) that codes for a specific protein can result in an abnormal protein that is unable to carry out its usual job.

The role of growth regulatory proteins in cell proliferation is analogous to the role of buttons on a blender that determine how fast the blender blades rotate, or if they rotate at all. It is when the usual precise regulation of cell growth is lost that cancer can occur. Cell division can get out of control when damage to specific genes in the cell's DNA results in abnormally functioning growth regulatory proteins. And although not all abnormal cell growth is malignant, it is this abnormal cell proliferation that sets up a situation in which cancer is possible.

In contrast to many cell types that have tough jobs and get worn out quickly, melanocytes have it easy. All they have to do is to make melanin. Because their job is simple, they live a long time and rarely if ever need to divide to replace themselves. In fact, when we cut ourselves deeply or have surgery in which deep layers of skin are removed (below the dermal-epidermal junction), resulting in removal of local melanocytes, the site of the skin removal remains nonpigmented because neighboring melanocytes do not divide to replace the melanocytes that were removed. This is why scars are almost always white.

When UV radiation from the sun or tanning booths damages one or more genes that regulate melanocyte cell division, the melanocytes may be able to proliferate, forming a cluster of cells, which appear on the skin as a mole. A mole is not dangerous and remains as a stable spot on the skin unless more genetic damage occurs in one of the melanocytes making up the mole. If enough damage occurs, a melanocyte may gain the ability to divide uncontrollably and even travel to other parts of the body. This is melanoma. Just how this happens and how you can detect the changes that may signal melanoma will be discussed in Chapters 2 and 4.

Nonmelanoma Skin Cancers

Besides melanoma, there are two other forms of skin cancer— **basal cell carcinoma** (BCC) and **squamous cell carcinoma** (SCC). BCCs and SCCs are more common and better known than melanoma. They both begin in the keratinocytes, not the melanocytes, and they behave very differently from melanoma. Because of their differences, it is best to think of skin cancer as either melanoma skin cancer or nonmelanoma skin cancer. Nonmelanoma skin cancers are the most common form of cancer in humans and occur primarily in fair-skinned Caucasians who have had extensive chronic sun exposure, especially outdoor workers such as farmers, dock workers, and construction workers. These skin cancers grow slowly and occur almost exclusively on sun-exposed parts of the body, most commonly the face and hands. BCCs are about four times more common than SCCs. They are typically the color of the surrounding skin, pink, or red with a shiny, slightly translucent appearance, and are often described as "pearly." They often contain a network of tiny blood vessels that can be seen easily on their surface and may result in bleeding with minor trauma. A central depression is also a commonly observed feature (see Plate 1). Occasionally, they are pigmented ("pigmented BCC") and may even resemble melanoma, but this is the exception rather than the rule.

SCCs (Plate 2) may have an appearance similar to BCCs (in fact, it is often difficult to distinguish between the two without a biopsy), but typically SCCs have a rougher surface, with scaling or crusting that may break open and bleed. Both BCCs and SCCs may appear to be sores on the skin that won't heal. While nonmelanoma skin cancers may be locally **invasive,** aggressive, and destructive (especially SCCs), they only rarely spread to other parts of the body. Once a BCC or SCC is removed, the patient can almost always be considered cured. However, persons who have had one BCC or SCC are at greater-than-average risk for the development of another. They are also at increased

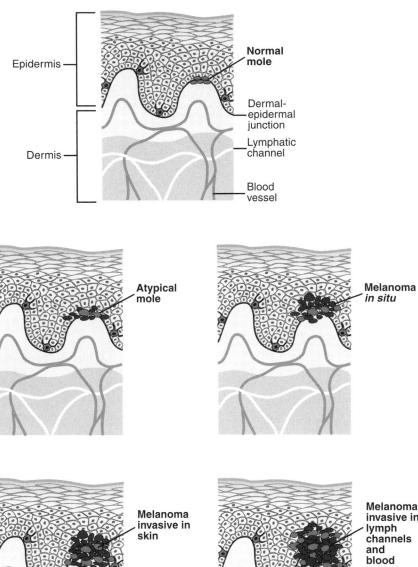

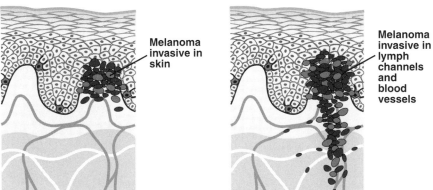

FIGURE 1.3. Progressive changes, from normal mole to invasive melanoma.

In the normal mole, the melanocytes are all similar in size and shape, and they form a symmetrically shaped pattern at the dermal-epidermal junction (Figure 1.3). In an atypical mole, the symmetry starts to disappear, and the cells become different in size and shape. These changes become increasingly pronounced as true melanoma develops and will be accompanied by progressive invasion of cells into the deeper layers of the skin, where the cells are able to invade the blood and lymphatic vessels.

How a small spot on the skin can become a life-threatening disease: progressive changes, as seen under the microscope, from a normal mole to an invasive melanoma

risk for the development of melanoma because both types of skin cancer are related to excessive sun exposure.

The most important difference between melanoma and non-melanoma skin cancers is that melanoma is much more likely to spread to the rest of the body. As noted above, this potential for spreading from the original cancer site is what makes melanoma so dangerous. Another way melanoma differs from nonmelanoma skin cancer is that it can originate in other areas of the body where the pigment-producing melanocytes are found. (Melanoma arising in these non-skin locations is uncommon and is discussed in more detail in Chapter 12.) Because melanoma arising in the skin is more common by far, when people speak of melanoma, they usually mean melanoma skin cancer. You may see it referred to as **cutaneous** malignant melanoma, however. *Cutaneous* is the medical term meaning "derived from or relating to the skin."

Because melanoma usually begins in existing moles on the skin, it is particularly important that we become familiar with the various pigmented spots on our skin. Chapter 2 describes these spots and which of them can develop into melanoma.

2

About Pigmented Lesions

Lesion is the medical term for any growth, benign or malignant, on the skin or other body organ. We all have a variety of colored (pigmented) lesions on our skin. Some we are born with (these are called **congenital** lesions); others arise as we get older (**acquired** lesions). Most of these spots are totally normal and should cause us no concern, but it is a good idea to become familiar with the pigmented lesions on our bodies, especially those that are brown or black, because changes in some of them can be the early signs of melanoma.

Five common types of **benign** (noncancerous) pigmented lesions of the skin are important because they may be precursors to melanoma or may be mistaken for melanoma. These are discussed in more detail below.

FRECKLES

Most people are able to recognize freckles (see Plate 3). They occur on sun-exposed sites of fair-skinned people and tend to wax and wane depending on the amount of recent sun exposure. After childhood, they often fade completely, particularly those located on the face. They are tan, completely flat, and almost always clumped together in large numbers. Freckles are caused by an increase in melanin production by normal melanocytes, not an increase in the number of melanocytes. Therefore, they have no risk of becoming melanoma themselves. People with a freckling tendency, however, do have a small increased risk for the development of melanoma (see Chapter 5).

Seborrheic Keratoses

A typical **seborrheic keratosis** is illustrated in Plate 4. Seborrheic keratoses are less well known than freckles, probably because they are rarely seen in people under the age of 40. They occur with increasing frequency with advancing age, however, and are quite common in middle-aged and elderly people of all skin types. They appear predominantly on the trunk and have a distinctive waxy, "stuck-on" appearance.

The average seborrheic keratosis is less than half an inch in diameter, although some are more than two inches across. They are most often different shades of grayish-brown or even black. Because seborrheic keratoses are large, raised, and, often, darkly pigmented, people are frequently concerned that they could be melanoma. They are derived from keratinocytes, however, not melanocytes, and so they never become melanoma. Fortunately, their distinctive appearance usually makes it possible to distinguish them on sight from moles or melanoma. Nevertheless, they often occur in large numbers, and it is important not to miss a melanoma hidden among a sea of seborrheic keratoses. If you have a number of seborrheic keratoses, you may want to ask your physician for a particularly careful skin examination to avoid missing a melanoma or melanoma precursor that may be hiding in the area.

Lentigos

Popularly known as "old age spots" or "liver spots," **lentigos** occur on sun-exposed sites mainly in older Caucasians. See Plate 5 for an example. Lentigos share many features with freckles: they are both completely flat, light brown or tan, and occur in fair-skinned Caucasians who have had a lot of sun exposure. They may also occur in lighter-skinned Asians—for example, Japanese people. Lentigos can almost always be distinguished from freckles, however. They are usually larger, they are isolated rather than clumped, and they do not wax and wane with the degree of recent sun exposure. Rather, they slowly increase in number and size with increasing age. They are present in 90% of Caucasians over the age of 60, although they may occur in younger people who have had excessive sun exposure. They are most common on the face, the back of the hands, and the forearms.

The most important way lentigos differ from freckles is that they are caused by a true increase in melanocyte number, rather than simply an increase in melanin production. As a result, lentigos can transform into melanoma (see Chapter 4 for more detail), just as moles can (see below).

Nevi

Nevus (plural, **nevi**) is the medical name for *mole*. We will use the words *nevus* and *mole* interchangeably, since you are likely to hear both terms. Nevi are clusters of melanocytes that appear as brown spots on the skin. Melanocytes that compose a nevus are usually called **nevus cells,** but they are really just melanocytes with some special characteristics. Virtually everyone has some moles; you need only look at your own skin for examples. Moles have many different appearances. They vary from person to person and from mole to mole on the same person. These differences and the reasons for them are discussed and illustrated below.

There are two broad categories of nevi: **common acquired nevi** and **congenital nevi**. Common acquired nevi are the most common type of pigmented skin lesion in humans. These moles are not present at the time of birth, but they are usually acquired in the early decades of life. The number present on any individual is determined by the person's age, cumulative sun exposure, and genetic predisposition. The average person has few or no moles in infancy and early childhood; the number increases with puberty, usually reaching a peak by age 30, after which age most people do not acquire new nevi. Furthermore, the moles that are present gradually disappear. Few elderly people have many moles. We do not know why moles follow this developmental cycle, but it probably relates at least in part to changes in the amount of sun exposure most of us experience as we get older. Most of us receive less intense sun exposure and fewer sunburns in the later decades of our lives than we do in childhood and the teenage years. Indeed, it has been estimated that we receive 80% of our lifetime sun exposure by age 18. Even though we all have moles, scientists believe that they serve no purpose, but are only the result of damage to melanocyte DNA.

Numerous lines of evidence have linked the development of moles to sun exposure, especially intense, intermittent sun exposure. The average number of nevi in Caucasian adults has been reported to be less than 25, but this number is growing with the lifestyle and clothing changes that are increasing our average lifetime sun exposure. It is probably now in the range of 30–35. Caucasians living in tropical or equatorial regions have a higher average number of moles than do Caucasians residing in temperate climates, and the vast majority of moles arise on parts of the body that have experienced intense, intermittent exposure to the sun.

But sun exposure is not the only factor involved in mole development. Some people who spend a great deal of time in the sun have hardly any nevi, while others with much less cumulative sun exposure have large numbers of moles. Just as we usually inherit our skin color and tendency (low or high) to develop freckles from one or both of our parents, it is clear that we also tend to inherit a higher or lower likelihood of developing moles. This is not to say that a person's tendency to develop nevi is always the same as that of her or his parents, but it frequently is. We will have more to say about this in the next chapter.

Why we believe that common acquired moles are the earliest step in the development of melanoma

There is strong evidence supporting this belief. The majority of melanomas arise from preexisting moles, and so the more moles you have, the greater your risk of developing melanoma. Also, scientists have been able to stimulate the growth of moles in animals by exposing them to known cancer-causing agents, or **carcinogens**. Finally, recently published data have demonstrated that most moles are clonal. This means that all the cells in the cluster are identical, indicating that they have all arisen from a single cell. The development of clonality is the earliest step in the development of cancer, for it suggests that the single cell has achieved a growth advantage over its neighboring cells, since it is dividing while they are not.

| *The majority of moles will never become melanoma* | If the average person in a population has 30–35 nevi and the lifetime risk of developing melanoma in the population is 1 in 100, then only 1 in 3,000–3,500 moles will ever become melanoma. In addition, some melanomas |

arise "anew" rather than from a preexisting mole, so this number represents an overestimate.

Most melanomas arise from moles, so the more moles you have, the greater your risk of developing melanoma. Fortunately, the likelihood that any given mole will ever become melanoma is very small.

Common Acquired Nevi

Common acquired nevi are subclassified as **junctional, intradermal,** or **compound.** These names derive from the location of clusters of melanocytes (nevus cells) that form the mole. Thus, in junctional nevi, the nevus cells are found at the skin's dermal-epidermal junction; in intradermal nevi, the nevus cells are in the dermis; and in compound nevi, there are nevus cells in both places. These three types of moles are illustrated in Figure 2.1. As they age, nevus cells divide more slowly, move down into the dermis, and make less pigment. Thus, the average nevus goes through a slow evolutionary progression over many years from a junctional nevus to a compound nevus and finally to an intradermal nevus that eventually disappears. This whole process generally occurs so slowly that we are unaware that it is going on.

With this evolutionary process in mind, you can understand why the three types of common acquired moles look different on the skin (Plate 6). Junctional nevi are flat because they contain relatively few cells. They are the darkest moles (medium to dark brown) because they are composed of the most immature nevus cells that are still able to produce large amounts of pigment. They are also closest to the surface of the skin. Compound nevi tend to be somewhat lighter shades of brown than junctional nevi due to decreased melanin production as the nevus cells age. They are often somewhat raised because they contain more nevus cells, which tend to push the epidermis up as they mi-

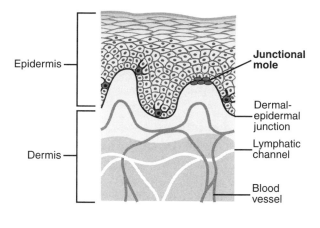

Epidermis —

Junctional mole

Dermal-epidermal junction

Dermis —

Lymphatic channel

Blood vessel

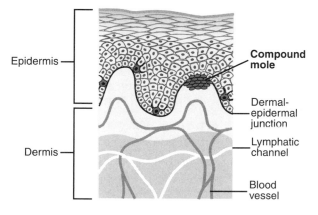

Epidermis —

Compound mole

Dermal-epidermal junction

Dermis —

Lymphatic channel

Blood vessel

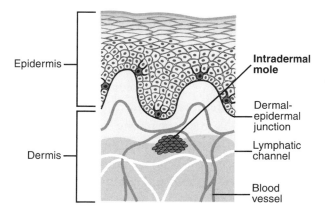

Epidermis —

Intradermal mole

Dermal-epidermal junction

Dermis —

Lymphatic channel

Blood vessel

FIGURE 2.1. The three types of common benign moles— junctional, compound, and intradermal. In junctional nevi (moles) the melanocytes (nevus cells) are confined to the dermal–epidermal junction. With compound nevi the nevus cells are both at the junction and in the dermis. In intradermal nevi the nevus cells are found only in the dermal layer of the skin. It is thought that there is a gradual progression from junctional nevi to intradermal nevi.

grate down into the dermis. Alternatively, they may have both a flat area and a raised area. The flat part is made up of junctional nevus cells, while the raised part is formed by intradermal cells. Intradermal nevi are more elevated and are often dome-shaped. They may contain so little pigment that they appear to be the same color as the surrounding skin.

It is not always possible to determine the subclassification of a nevus by looking at it on the skin; to be certain, it must be removed and examined under a microscope. If you have a mole removed, your doctor's report should classify the nevus as junctional, intradermal, or compound. Mole type is important because most melanomas are thought to arise from junctional nevi (or the junctional component of compound nevi). Thus, the moles you should watch most closely for change are the flat ones or the ones with a flat component. The changes that you should be looking for will be discussed in detail in Chapter 4. It may seem surprising that it is usually junctional moles or the junctional part of compound moles that become melanoma. After all, it is the intradermal moles that extend into the dermis where the blood vessels and lymphatics are. Junctional moles can become melanoma because the nevus cells in junctional moles are young, and only young and actively dividing cells have the capacity to become malignant. Once they have become cancerous, they may then invade down into the dermis and into the local blood vessels or lymphatics. (Benign intradermal nevus cells do not have the ability to invade blood vessels or lymphatic channels.)

Congenital Nevi

Congenital nevi is the medical term for moles that are present from birth. Popularly known as "birthmarks," they occur in 1 in 100 newborns in all races. Occasionally more than one may be present. They usually last for life and do not go through the normal aging process that most acquired moles go through. Sometimes, though, they are "attacked" by the immune system and disappear, leaving behind a white area with no pigment. Congenital nevi have a distinct appearance under the microscope, wrapping themselves around nerves, blood vessels, hair follicles, and sweat glands so that a **pathologist** (a doctor who studies the microscopic changes in tissues caused by disease) can usually tell a mole is congenital even without knowing that the patient has had it since birth. Congenital nevi tend to be larger than acquired nevi, most commonly one-half inch to an inch in diameter, though they may be very large (see the discussion of giant congenital nevi below). They range in color from tan to brown to nearly black and may have any appearance, but typically they contain hair and have a pebbly raised surface with stippled or dotted pigmentation (Plate 7). They may also have irregular borders, which along with their often variable pigmentation and large size may make them resemble melanoma. They can easily be distinguished from melanoma, however, simply by knowing that the mole has looked the same since birth. It is important to realize that melanoma can arise from congenital moles and that, like acquired junctional and compound nevi, congenital moles need to be monitored closely for any change.

There has been much controversy as to whether or not congenital moles are more likely to develop into melanoma than common acquired nevi. Most researchers agree, however, that the larger the mole, the greater the risk of developing melanoma. The best and most recent data have shown that congenital moles smaller than three-quarters of an inch are not at much higher risk of developing into melanoma than common acquired nevi. They do not need to be removed, therefore, unless they are in a difficult-to-observe place or have features that make it difficult to see if they are changing. Changes in dark-colored moles or those with spotty pigmentation, for example, may be difficult to notice. An alternative to removal in this case is to take a photograph of the mole to make it easier to detect any change that may occur. You may also choose to have a small congenital mole removed if it is in a place that has received a lot of intense sun exposure in the past. Congenital moles that are larger than three-quarters of an inch are more likely to develop melanoma and should be completely removed if feasible. Again, the bigger the mole, the greater the risk.

Giant congenital (or "bathing trunk") **nevi** are an unusual type of congenital nevus. They are very large moles often found on the back and buttocks, in what has been described as a bathing trunk distribution. They may extend into the anus and may penetrate into the muscle below the skin. They may also penetrate into the covering around the brain or spinal cord (**leptomeninges**). They occur in 1 in 100,000 births and affect both sexes and all races. In rare cases, they may be inherited. Giant congenital nevi may be small (1–2 inches across) or very large, covering up to 25% of the skin's surface. They are dark brown or bluish-black and tend to have a raised, pebbly surface covered with black hair. As you might imagine, the larger ones are usually of cosmetic concern to parents, and later to the child. There is a 5–10% lifetime risk that large giant congenital nevi will develop into melanoma. Half of these melanomas will develop in childhood. Because they are very large and penetrate the skin very deeply (often into underlying muscle), their complete removal is usually not feasible. Laser treatment is ineffective for the same reasons. The best option for most is therefore to watch these moles closely for any change that may suggest transformation to melanoma, and to remove any worrisome areas. This is possible because when melanoma does arise in a giant congenital nevus, it begins in a very localized part of the lesion. We will talk more about giant congenital nevi in Chapter 12.

Although only moles and lentigos can develop into melanomas, other skin lesions, such as freckles, are associated with skin types that are more vulnerable than others to the development of melanoma. We will discuss these risk factors later in the book. Meanwhile, in the next chapter we will look at the way acquired moles form and how they can become cancerous. We will also discuss why there has been such an increase in cases of melanoma over the last few decades.

3

What Causes Melanoma, and
Why Are So Many People Getting It?

A great deal of the sun's energy that reaches the earth does so as visible light, commonly called sunlight. Some of the sun's rays, however, have wavelengths too short to be visible to the human eye. There are two types of invisible rays, or radiation: *infrared radiation*, which brings the sun's heat to earth, and *ultraviolet radiation*, or *ultraviolet light*.

Ultraviolet (UV) light is essential for life because it is used by plants to generate their energy (and in turn, of course, people and animals generate much of their energy from plants). But the UV rays are also the rays that cause sunburns, skin cancer, and aging. Although we can't see it, UV light penetrates our bodies through our skin and our eyes.

There are three kinds of ultraviolet light: UVA, UVB, and UVC. No UVC rays reach the surface of the earth because they are absorbed by the ozone layer surrounding the earth. UVB rays cause the burning that you see and feel after spending time in the sun; they can also cause aging and skin cancers. UVA rays penetrate more deeply into the skin than UVB rays, and evidence is mounting to suggest that UVA rays also cause aging and, most importantly, skin cancer, including melanoma. That is why, in Chapter 6, we recommend you use sunscreen that is labeled UVA/UVB—so that it offers some protection from both of these kinds of UV light. (You may have noticed that suntan booths advertise that they use UVA rays, touting them as "safe" for tanning. But we now know that UVA rays, once thought to be harmless, can actually cause a great deal of skin damage also, including cancer.)

In the right amounts and at the right wavelengths, UV radiation is beneficial (see "Benefits of UV radiation," below), but there is compelling evidence that overexposure to UV radiation is by far the leading cause of melanoma.

Here are the facts:

1. Melanoma occurs primarily on parts of the body that receive intense intermittent exposure to the sun. (We'll discuss this further in Chapter 5.)

2. The overwhelming majority of melanomas develop in Caucasians, whose melanocytes produce smaller amounts and lighter forms of melanin than do those of naturally dark-skinned people, providing them with less protection against the sun.

3. Data from a variety of studies show a correlation between increasing recreational sun exposure over the past 50 years and the increasing incidence of melanoma in the population.

4. The incidence of melanoma in any given geographical area increases proportionately with the region's yearly amount of UV exposure.

5. Population migration studies have demonstrated that when people residing in temperate climates with a relatively low incidence of melanoma migrate to tropical climates with a higher incidence of melanoma, their risk of melanoma increases.

Benefits of UV radiation

In modest amounts, UV radiation is important to our health. It stimulates our bodies to produce vitamin D, which allows us to absorb the calcium we need to build and maintain strong bones and teeth. Because of its bacteria-killing properties, UV light of the proper wavelength is used to sterilize operating rooms and surgical instruments, and UV radiation is used in conjunction with drugs for treating the skin condition psoriasis. Babies born with a condition known as jaundice, in which their livers are not able to rid their bodies of a substance called bilirubin, are treated with ultraviolet light either artificially or by being placed in sunny windows. The UV light converts the bilirubin to a form the babies' bodies can get rid of. A buildup of bilirubin in the liver can cause brain damage and even death, and thousands of babies are saved each year by this treatment.

In recent decades physicians and scientists have learned a great deal about how cancer develops. The study of known melanoma risk factors, particularly excessive sun exposure, and the study of the genes of families in which melanoma seems to be hereditary have given them a better understanding of how melanoma cancers develop.

THE MULTIPLE HIT THEORY

The most widely accepted theory about how cancer develops is known as the *multiple hit theory*. According to this theory, in order for a cell to become cancerous, several of the genes that regulate cell growth must be damaged (or "hit"). Damage to a smaller number of these genes or to less important genes results in a **premalignant** cell rather than a full-blown cancer cell. When one of the regulatory genes of a melanocyte is damaged—say, by ultraviolet radiation from the sun or a tanning booth—the cell's "brakes" are loosened a bit, and it is able to divide and proliferate, when ordinarily it would not. This is thought to be how moles are formed and explains why they almost always arise on parts of the body that are exposed to UV radiation.

When a cell divides, the new cell is an exact duplicate, or **clone,** of the original cell (see Figure 3.1). Its DNA is identical to the DNA of the parent cell. Thus, the damaged gene that allowed the cell to divide in the first place gets passed along to all of the cells subsequently produced by the parent cell. If another regulatory gene is later damaged in any of the melanocytes composing a mole, the DNA of the cells arising from this "double-hit" cell will also have this additional damage. If enough regulatory genes are mutated, melanoma may eventually result. It is not known exactly how many genes and which combination or combinations of genes must be damaged in a melanocyte for melanoma to result, but we do know that cells with one "hit" to their DNA are more likely than normal cells to sustain further DNA mutations.

There appears to be a *continuum* from a normal cell to a cancerous cell, with increasing malignant potential resulting from an increasing number of "hits." Moles are thought to represent the earliest step in the continuum of melanoma development, with subsequent steps including the progression to an atypical mole, then to **melanoma *in situ*** ("in place"), and eventually to **invasive** mel-

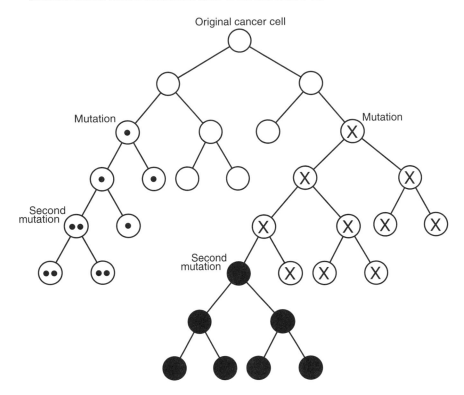

FIGURE 3.1. As normal cells divide, mutations do occur, although rarely. When this happens, all of the daughter cells that arise from this mutated cell contain the same mutation (they are identical) and are defined as clones. Cells with one mutation are more prone to the development of further mutations as they proliferate than are normal cells. Each mutation is different, resulting in a "mixed" population of tumor cells—one with multiple different clones. This is one of the major reasons why advanced cancer is so difficult to treat: it only takes one clone that is not killed by the treatment to prevent a cure, because that clone can continue to proliferate (and mutate).

anoma. In melanoma in situ, the cells have become cancerous but the cancer is confined to the dermal-epidermal junction and has not yet invaded the dermis. Melanoma in situ is sometimes called *radial growth phase melanoma* or *noninvasive melanoma*. The development from a mole to melanoma in situ is gradual, taking months or

---

	Clark's Levels

In 1967, Dr. Wallace Clark established a system for categorizing melanomas according to how deeply they had invaded the skin. He assigned numerical levels to the different layers of skin, as illustrated by Fig. 3.2. Level I represents melanoma confined to the dermal-epidermal junction (melanoma in situ). Level II melanoma has invaded beyond the dermal-epidermal junction into the papillary dermis; level III melanoma completely fills the papillary dermis; level IV melanoma invades into the reticular dermis; and level V represents invasion into the subcutaneous fat or deeper.

This system is still used today to help grade the severity of a melanoma and its likelihood of eventually spreading from its site of origin.

---

even years. In contrast, once the mole's cells have become malignant, the spread of melanoma is unpredictable; it can continue its slow pace or it can be quite rapid.

ABOUT INVASIVE MELANOMA

Once melanoma cells have invaded the dermis, they can enter the lymphatic system and bloodstream and in this way travel throughout the body. This is why a small spot on the skin can lead to serious illness and even death. The spread of cancer cells is known as **metastasis.** In order for a melanoma cell to metastasize, it must adhere to the wall of the blood or lymphatic vessel, travel to a new location, penetrate through the vessel, and then grow in the liver, brain, lungs, or wherever it is adapted to survive. Most melanoma cells do not have the ability to do this, but it takes only one cell with this ability to allow metastasis to occur.

The likelihood that a melanoma lesion has metastasized is directly related to how deeply it has invaded the skin. We will discuss this in more detail later in the book. For now, though, it is important to note that since **Clark's level** I melanoma is confined to the dermal-epidermal junction, it is not considered invasive, because there are no blood or lymphatic vessels in the epidermis. (See the description of Clark's levels, above.) When we use the term *invasive melanoma,* we

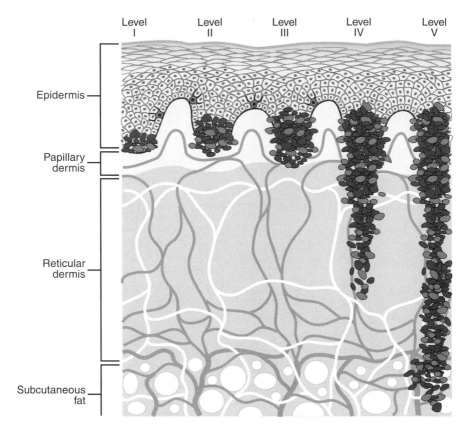

FIGURE 3.2. Representation of Clark's levels of invasion. Most melanomas develop at the dermal-epidermal junction and, if confined there, are called level I, or melanoma in situ. The melanoma cells then grow progressively downward with time. The deeper the growth, the greater the likelihood of spread beyond the skin. In level II, the melanoma cells have invaded into the upper (papillary) dermis. In level III, the melanoma cells completely fill the papillary dermis. In level IV, the melanoma cells have invaded the second layer of the dermis (the reticular dermis), and in level V the melanoma cells have invaded the fat under the skin. The risk of recurrence of melanoma is directly correlated with how deeply the melanoma cells invade the skin.

The concept of metastases frequently leads to confusion. It is sometimes thought that a person with widely metastatic melanoma has, for example, brain cancer, lung cancer, and liver cancer, in addition to melanoma. This is not the case. The patient only has one type of cancer—in this case, melanoma—but it has invaded different body organs. Melanoma in the brain is still melanoma and can be identified as such when sample cells are examined under a microscope. Melanoma cells are cancerous melanocytes and retain the characteristics of melanocytes wherever they are found. Cancer that arises initially in the brain (or true brain cancer) and melanoma look completely different from each other under the microscope, because brain cancer arises from brain cells rather than from melanocytes. The same is true of lung cancer, which arises from lung cells, or liver cancer, which arises from liver cells, and so on.

Frequent misconceptions about metastases

mean that the melanoma cells have invaded down into the dermis. This does not necessarily mean that the melanoma has metastasized because invasion into the dermal or even subcutaneous layers of the skin can occur without invasion into the blood vessels or lymphatics.

THE RISING INCIDENCE OF MELANOMA

The incidence of melanoma has been rising in Caucasian populations since approximately the 1940s. Initially, the rise was slow and hardly noticeable, but recently it has become frighteningly fast. Currently, melanoma is the most rapidly increasing malignancy in Caucasians throughout the world, and in high-risk populations it has reached what medical journals have termed epidemic proportions. Before 1940, melanoma was an uncommon disease. The lifetime risk for Caucasians in the United States in 1935 was only 1 in 1,500. By 1996, the lifetime risk in the same population had risen to 1 in 87, and the estimated risk by the year 2000 is 1 in 70.

Alarmingly, in the United States this escalating incidence shows no sign of leveling off (see Figure 3.3). Furthermore, the U.S. data almost certainly represent a significant underestimate of the true inci-

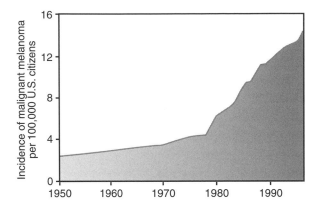

FIGURE 3.3. Rising annual incidence of malignant melanoma (number of cases per year per 100,000 population) in the United States between 1950 and 1995. Note the steep rise in the number of cases beginning about 1980 and continuing until the present time.

dence of melanoma. This is because U.S. registries that collect statistics about cancer are hospital-based, so patients not seen in a hospital are never reported to the registry. This means that many patients are not counted in the statistics because they have early or thin melanomas requiring no treatment other than surgical excision of the lesion in a doctor's office. Given their excellent prognosis, most of these patients will never have their melanoma treated in a hospital. A recent study that surveyed community physicians in the United States about the number of patients in their practice diagnosed with melanoma indicated that the real incidence of the disease is two or three times the number reported by the registries.

A dramatic increase in the incidence of melanoma in Caucasian populations similar to that seen in the United States has been reported across the globe over the past few decades. The incidence has remained unchanged or has increased only slightly in non-Caucasian populations over similar time periods. In Australia, where the incidence of melanoma is the highest in the world, the lifetime risk of invasive melanoma (Clark's levels II–V) in 1998 was 1 in 30 for the entire population. In 1998, the lifetime risk of developing melanoma in Queensland (one of the Australian states closest to the equator) was 1 in 15.

In fact, melanoma is currently the most common malignancy in males aged 25–59 years in Australia and is the second most common malignancy (after breast cancer) in females in the same age group, as well as in both males and females in the 15- to 24-year-old age group.

In most Australian states, every diagnosis of invasive melanoma is required to be reported to cancer registries, regardless of whether the patient is seen in the hospital or in a clinic. Thus, the Australian figures represent a more accurate assessment of melanoma incidence than do the U.S. data. Even in Australia, however, melanoma in situ (Clark's level I) is not included in the incidence data. If it were, the numbers would nearly double.

Although the overall incidence of melanoma in Australia continues to rise, the rate of increase is slowing, particularly in women; and in the youngest age groups, it is even decreasing. This is a tribute

Is there a real increase in the incidence of melanoma, or is it just reported more accurately now?

The trend toward earlier diagnosis has led some people to speculate that the reports of increased incidence of melanoma are artificially high due to a heightened awareness and earlier diagnosis. Several pieces of evidence demonstrate that this is not the case—that the reports reflect a real increase in the incidence of the disease.

First, while thin lesions account for most of the increased incidence of melanoma, the incidence of thick lesions has not decreased with time, as would be expected if the growing number of cases were simply a result of earlier diagnosis. Second, because of its nature, melanoma that is not diagnosed when thin will eventually demand the attention of the patient. If the increase in melanoma cases were merely the result of earlier diagnosis, it would mean that in the past a great number of people developed melanoma that was never diagnosed or that went away. Unfortunately, this isn't possible. Melanoma doesn't just sit there; eventually, if left alone, it kills.

Finally, despite the fact that more and more people are being diagnosed at early stages and have an excellent chance of surviving the disease, the number of people dying from melanoma each year continues to rise. The only explanation for this increasing death rate in the face of increased early diagnosis is an even faster increase in incidence.

to impressive educational campaigns about the causes and prevention of melanoma that Australia instituted in the 1960s.

WHAT IS CAUSING THIS "EPIDEMIC" OF MELANOMA?

Melanoma is largely a disease of the modern lifestyle. The rapid rise in melanoma incidence we are observing is due to dramatic changes in this century in the way people spend their time and the kind of clothes they wear. Combined with modern attitudes toward suntanning, these changes have resulted in a significant increase in our lifetime sun exposure.

At the turn of the twentieth century, most people did outdoor work such as farming, construction, and shipping. Technology was so limited that, except for the wealthy, few people had what we would call leisure time. Food for the family's table was usually grown at home and had to be prepared from scratch, without the modern-day conveniences of prepared foods, microwave ovens, freezers, or fast food restaurants. Clothing was made and washed by hand, and people traveled on foot or by horse and buggy. The upper classes considered pale skin fashionable; it distinguished them from common outdoor laborers. Women of fashion wore long dresses, carried parasols, and used special cosmetics, all to achieve the palest skin possible. Fashionable men considered short sleeves and short pants sissified; instead, they wore suits or long pants and long-sleeved shirts (Figure 3.4).

Twentieth-century technology changed this dramatically. Farmwork and other outdoor jobs were increasingly mechanized and required fewer laborers. As a result of increasing industrialization and urbanization, the majority of the labor force moved inside. Pale skin became the norm. You might think that as workers moved inside, the incidence of skin cancer would diminish, but other factors were at work: The work year for factory and office workers included vacations, and such household appliances as refrigerators, gas stoves, and vacuum cleaners began to simplify home life. Leisure time became an important sign of prosperity, and more and more of that time came to be spent outdoors.

In the 1920s, for example, only the wealthy traveled to exclusive beachside resorts. Gradually, they were joined by a growing middle class with leisure time and money for travel. Recently there has been

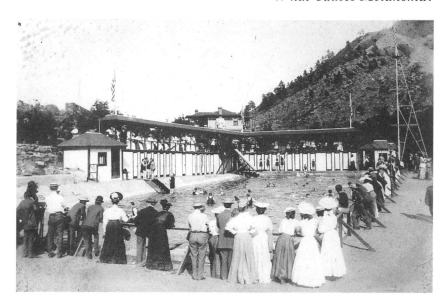

FIGURE 3.4. Fashions from the early twentieth century. "Sunbathers" at a community swimming pool, Colorado, 1917.

a virtual explosion in the number of tropical island resorts and in the number of people able to afford to travel to them. The travel sections of major newspapers are filled with ads for vacation specials priced to allow a growing number of people to spend at least two weeks in the sun. In addition, retiring to the warmth of Florida or Arizona is no longer possible only for the rich. At the same time, the fitness boom has sent droves of people outdoors, running, walking, swimming, rollerblading, and bicycling. Many people consider having a tan (especially in winter) chic, attractive, and a sign of prosperity and good health. We now know that the advent of sunny vacations, bikinis, shorts, and tanning salons set the stage for the epidemic we are now witnessing. Figure 3.3 illustrates what has happened to the incidence of melanoma with the introduction of specific lifestyle and clothing changes.

Given the lifestyle and clothing changes described above, it has been surprising to find that, despite also having an association with excessive sun exposure, the incidence of nonmelanoma skin cancer has

| What about the ozone layer? | A lot has been written about holes in the ozone layer and their effect on the amount of UV radiation reaching the earth. The ozone layer filters out much of the damaging |

rays of the sun, particularly UVB and UVC rays. Holes in the ozone layer have been particularly noted over the Southern Hemisphere and appear to be the result of chemicals (chlorofluorocarbons, or CFCs) released into the atmosphere from sources like the aerosols in spray cans and refrigerants used in air conditioning. There is, however, very little evidence that these holes have led to an increase in UV radiation that can be measured on earth. Also, the rise in the incidence of melanoma is unlikely to be due to a decrease in ozone. There is usually a long latent period (20–30 years) between intense sun exposure and the development of melanoma; changes in the ozone layer have been noted only over the past 10–15 years. Thus, while depletion of ozone may make some contribution to the current problem of melanoma, at present it is minor compared to the changes in lifestyle that have occurred over the past 50 years. There is, however, little doubt that continued depletion of the ozone layer, if not curbed, may be an important factor in the future.

increased far more slowly than the incidence of melanoma. Nonmelanoma skin cancer is still far more common than melanoma, but the rate at which people get it has not grown nearly as quickly. This is probably because most of the increased sun exposure we now receive is *intense and intermittent.* Researchers now believe that this kind of exposure is a more potent risk factor for the development of melanoma, while nonmelanoma skin cancer is more closely linked to *chronic* sun exposure. Most moles, and most melanomas, arise on parts of the body that have been exposed to high doses of intermittent sun, such as the back and the legs. Moles and melanoma are uncommon on the hands and face, even though these areas are usually the most sun-exposed parts of people's bodies. So, people who work indoors 50 weeks a year and have fun in the sun 2 weeks a year, and on some weekends, may be seriously increasing their chances of developing melanoma (more on this in Chapter 5).

Unfortunately, U.S. surveys as recent as 1994 have demonstrated that despite knowing about the perils of sun exposure, which include

Australia has the highest incidence of melanoma in the world. The racial makeup of the population and the geography of the country are important factors in this. Most of the non-Aboriginal population originated in northern European countries, where sunlight is scarce and skin is fair. Until 1973, a racially biased immigration policy allowed only whites into the country, so that the fair-skinned European stock has not been "diluted out" by interbreeding with darker-skinned people. Sun is hardly scarce in Australia, particularly in the northern states closest to the equator. In addition, because the center of the country is desert, all of the major cities in Australia line the coasts, and they all have sunny beaches. Along with lifestyle and clothing fashions, these conditions have led to an explosive growth in the number of cases of melanoma.

Why is there so much melanoma in Australia?

a dramatic acceleration of skin aging in addition to melanoma and nonmelanoma skin cancers, many people continue to spend hours in the sun in skimpy clothing. Clearly, it will be difficult to change the modern lifestyle. It is hard to imagine people wearing long-sleeved shirts and pants while jogging on a hot day or giving up their vacations in lush tropical resorts. Nevertheless, it is encouraging that the incidence of melanoma in the younger age groups in Australia, where educational campaigns have been most extensive, has begun to decline. This suggests that modest lifestyle changes such as avoiding peak sunlight hours and regular use of sunscreens, hats, and other protective clothing can have an impact on this potentially fatal disease. (For details on melanoma prevention, see Chapter 6.)

DO GENES AFFECT A PERSON'S CHANCES OF DEVELOPING MELANOMA?

Although most melanomas are associated with the sun's UV radiation, not everyone who has spent time unprotected in direct sunlight gets melanoma. It is also true that melanomas sometimes occur in people who have no history of excessive sun exposure, and it appears on parts of the body that have not been exposed to the sun and among people with dark skin. In rare families, a propensity to develop melanoma is hereditary. We have much more to learn about what causes melanoma and how it develops, and research is ongoing. One area that is being studied is genetics. Researchers have been studying the genes that regulate melanocyte proliferation and the genetic profiles of families in which the tendency to develop melanoma seems to be inherited.

One of the regulatory genes that serves as a "brake" or an "off" button to inhibit melanocyte proliferation is the p16 gene. It was the first gene shown to be involved in the development of melanoma. The p16 gene is a member of the class of genes known as **tumor suppressor genes.** The major role of tumor suppressor genes is not to suppress tumors that have already formed (as the name suggests) but, rather, to precisely regulate the proliferation of normal cells. When all of the genes responsible for regulating the proliferation of a particular cell type are present and functioning properly, cell division is well controlled and occurs only when the body has a demand for that cell type. When one or more of these genes is damaged or absent, however, cell division is able to proceed in a more haphazard, poorly regulated fashion, resulting in the production of cells the body does not need. Melanocytes are one of the major cell types in the body whose growth is controlled by the p16 gene (other cell types rely on different regulatory genes), and melanoma is the most common malignancy in people with a p16 mutation. People with a p16 mutation are also at an increased risk for pancreatic cancer and a specific type of benign brain tumor called a meningioma, but these tumors are much less common.

Genes that control melanocyte growth may be damaged by sunlight. They may also be inherited in an abnormal form, or rarely, they may even be absent. Such an inherited genetic defect is known as a **germline mutation,** because the mutation is present in the sperm or egg cell (the so-called germ cells) at the time of conception and subsequently gets passed along to *every* cell in the body as the fetus develops. Since cells with one "hit" are at increased risk for acquiring further "hits," virtually everyone with a germline mutation of one p16 gene in every melanocyte in his or her body will, given sun exposure, eventually develop melanoma: it is only a matter of time. Not surprisingly, such people frequently develop melanoma at a young

Following the fundamental research first reported in 1989 demonstrating a link between the p16 gene and melanoma, researchers in Melbourne, Australia, studied a family with a history of melanoma. All of the family members with melanoma who have had their blood tested have been shown to have a specific defect in one of their two copies of the p16 gene, while those who have never developed melanoma have two normal copies of the p16 gene. Because the *same defect* was found in all of the affected family members, we know a germline mutation is involved, rather than one that has been acquired. (There are many different ways the p16 gene—or any gene, for that matter—can be mutated.)

A family with a hereditary tendency toward melanoma

Parents, children, and siblings of affected members in this family could undergo genetic testing to determine whether or not they carry a defective p16 gene. Because germline mutations affect every cell in the body, a small blood sample is all that is needed for testing. Those testing positive for a defective p16 gene will be at very high risk for the development of melanoma. They should take every precaution to avoid UV damage and should be especially vigilant for early signs that melanoma is developing (see Chapter 4). Those who test negative will have a risk similar to that of the rest of the population.

age—in their 20s or 30s—and they often develop more than one **primary** melanoma. (A primary melanoma is the cluster of cancerous melanocytes that appears on the skin.)

People born with a damaged or absent p16 gene often have several close relatives who have had one or more melanomas. Many other family members will go on to develop melanoma at some point in their lives, as they acquire more damage to their already abnormal melanocyte DNA. Indeed, it was the study of such families with multiple members with melanoma that led to the discovery of the role of the p16 gene in melanoma in 1989.

An **acquired mutation** is one in which the genetic damage occurs later in life in a single cell (for example, UV-induced damage to the p16 gene of a single melanocyte) so that only nevus cells subsequently arising from the defective melanocyte will carry the mutation. People with acquired mutations cannot pass them on to their offspring unless the new mutation happens to occur in a germ cell. (New mutations can occur in the germ cells by chance, but they are not known to result from UV damage.)

Just as genetic testing is now available for genes linked to hereditary breast and colon cancer, a few centers are now able to screen people with a strong family history of melanoma for missing or defective copies of the p16 gene. This test is currently being used primarily for research, but it will almost certainly become more widely available for patient testing in the near future. Because p16 is only one of the genes involved the development of melanoma, however, this test will be of only limited use, even to members of families with a history of melanoma. We know there are other important genes involved in the development of melanoma because members of most families with hereditary melanoma are born with two normal copies of the p16 gene.[1] Scientists have narrowed down the chromosomal location of some of these other genes, but the exact genes themselves have not yet been identified.

. . .

In this chapter, we saw how the multiple hit theory explains how repeated bombardment of a melanocyte's DNA by UV radiation can allow the cell to begin the uncontrolled proliferation that characterizes melanoma. We learned that genetic studies have helped explain why some people seem to be more vulnerable to melanoma than others. In Chapters 4 and 5, we will see what changes in moles and lentigos to watch out for and how we can assess our own personal risk of developing melanoma.

---

[1]We all have two copies of every gene. One is inherited from our mother; the other is inherited from our father.

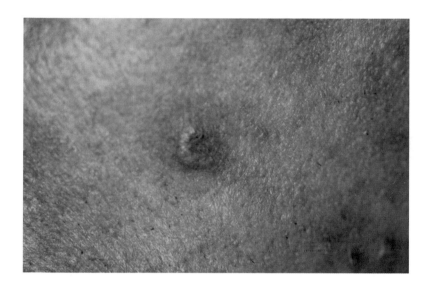

PLATE 1. Basal cell carcinoma (BCC). BCCs are often raised off the skin, scaly, and slightly pink. They may be pale and shiny, with a pearly appearance, or appear as a sore that will not heal. They grow slowly and occur most commonly on the face, neck, and upper torso. By permission of Anti-Cancer Council of Victoria.

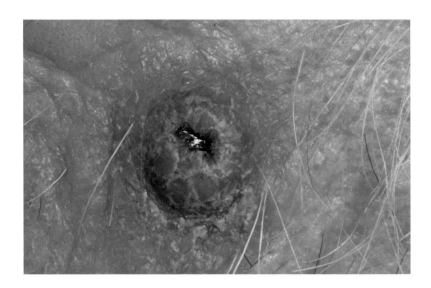

PLATE 2. Squamous cell carcinoma (SCC). SCCs are thickened, red, scaly lesions, often with a crater-like center. They are found on parts of the body most often exposed to the sun. They may appear as a sore that will not heal, and they grow slowly over several months. It can be difficult to distinguish SCCs from BCCs without a biopsy, but SCCs tend to be scalier and redder than BCCs. By permission of Anti-Cancer Council of Victoria.

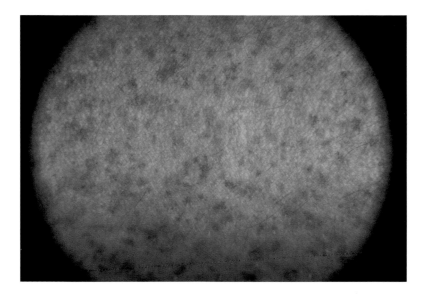

Plate 3. Freckles. Small, flat, and ranging from tan to brown in color, freckles are usually clumped together so closely that they are impossible to count. They occur most often on parts of the body receiving the most sun exposure. They may wax and wane in density of color with the amount of recent sun exposure. Lentigos have a similar appearance but are usually larger, more isolated, and do not darken and lighten according to length of sun exposure. By permission of Anti-Cancer Council of Victoria.

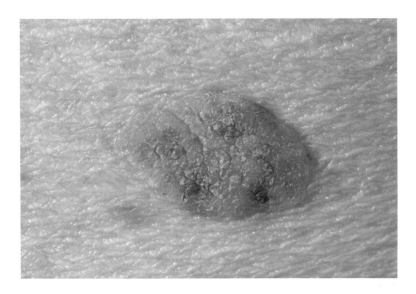

Plate 4. Seborrheic keratosis. Note the classic, raised, "stuck-on" appearance and the waxy, scaly surface as well as the large size. (This lesion was 1 centimeter in its longest dimension.) Seborrheic keratoses may vary in color from gray to any shade of brown to nearly black. By permission of Anti-Cancer Council of Victoria.

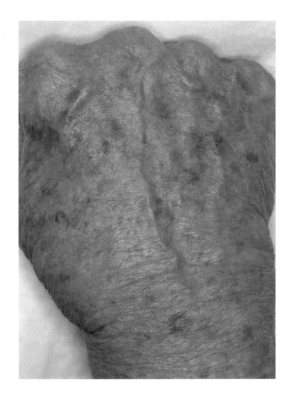

PLATE 5. Multiple lentigos on the hand of a woman 70 years old. Lentigos are also called "old age spots" or "liver spots." They are very common in Caucasians, especially on the hands, forearms, and face. They increase in number with advancing age. Like moles, they should be watched for signs of change because they, too, can develop into melanoma.

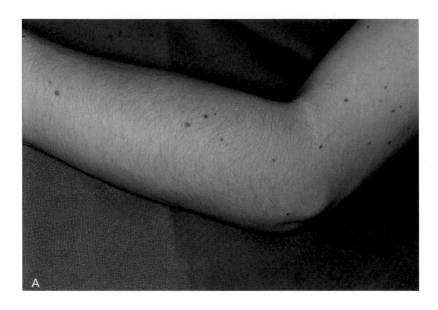

PLATE 6. *A*, Multiple small, flat (junctional) moles. All of these appear completely benign: they are small and have regular borders and uniform color. *B*, Two benign compound nevi. Both have raised centers with flat, regular borders. There are two parts to these moles: a junctional (flat) component and an intradermal (raised) component—thus, the name *compound nevi*. *C*, Benign intradermal nevus. This is a round, usually raised mole with uniform color, regular borders, and nearly perfect symmetry. Often these moles are less darkly pigmented than junctional or compound nevi because the melanocytes in the mole move into the lower layers of the skin and produce less melanin, but benign intradermal nevi vary greatly in appearance from person to person. Generally, lighter-skinned people have lighter-colored nevi. This person has olive-colored skin. By permission of Anti-Cancer Council of Victoria.

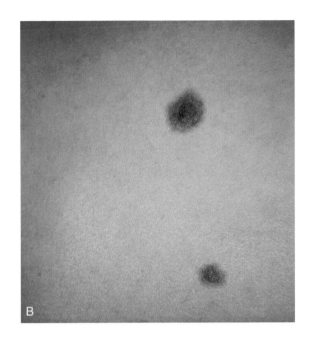

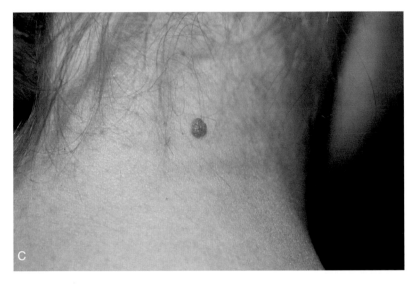

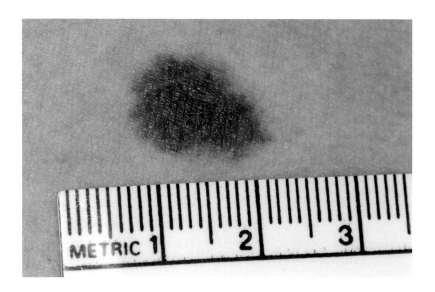

PLATE 7. Congenital nevus. If this person's medical history weren't available, this lesion would be cause for concern: it might be an atypical mole or even melanoma because of its large size, slight asymmetry, indistinct and irregular margins, and color variegation. But since the nevus has been present, without change, from the time the person was born, it needs only careful watching. The stippled or dotted pigmentation is typical for congenital moles, but they may look very different from this, too. Congenital moles larger than 2 centimeters have been associated with an increased risk of melanoma, and removal of these larger moles should be strongly considered.

The ABCDs of Melanoma

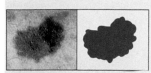

Asymmetry — One half doesn't match the other half.

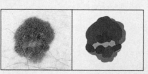

Color — The pigmentation is not uniform. Shades of tan, brown and black are present. Dashes of red, white and blue add to the mottled appearance.

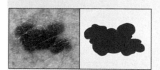

Border irregularity — The edges are ragged, notched or blurred.

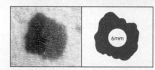

Diameter — greater than six millimeters (about the size of a pencil eraser). Any growth of a mole should be of concern.

PLATE 8. ABCD criteria.

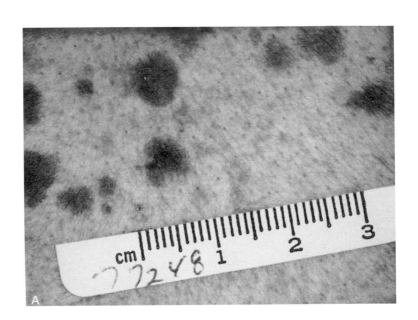

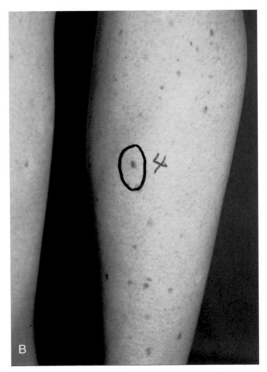

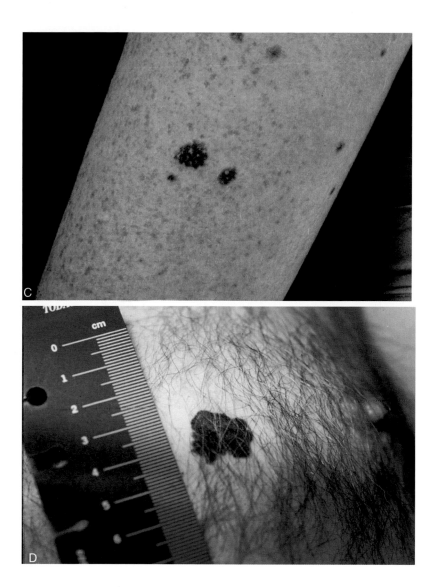

PLATE 9. *A, B, C,* Three different examples of dyplastic nevi. *D,* Melanoma. This is a classic melanoma, because it has all of the ABCD characteristics: note the asymmetry, the notched, very irregular borders, the color variegation, and the large size. Surprisingly, this lesion was only a Clark's level II, 0.56 Breslow depth, which illustrates the concept that the appearance on the skin (which in this case suggests a more deeply invasive lesion) does not always correlate with the microscopic appearance. However, this is true in reverse, as well: the lesion may appear more benign on the skin than it does when examined under a microscope. By permission of Anti-Cancer Council of Victoria.

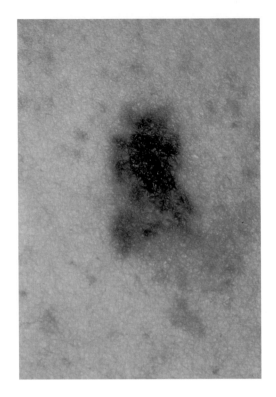

PLATE 10. Another melanoma meeting all four ABCD criteria.

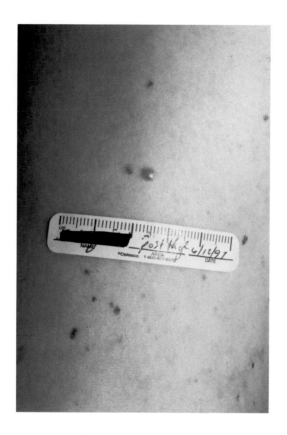

PLATE 11. Amelanotic melanoma. The completely nonpigmented lesion shown here among several benign-appearing nevi was initially thought by the patient to be a bug bite. When it failed to clear up after several months, however, it was removed and found to be an amelanotic melanoma. The diagnosis of amelanotic melanoma cannot be made without a biopsy. Just looking at this lesion, one might think that it is a BCC or a benign intradermal nevus. Just like pigmented melanomas, amelanotic melanomas may have many different appearances.

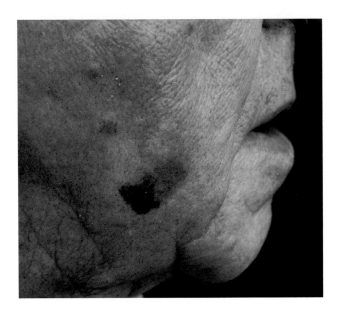

PLATE 12. Lentigo maligna melanoma on the face. Lentigo maligna melanoma is one of the forms of melanoma that develops most often in older people, especially on the face. It begins as a flat brown "age spot" (lentigo). Lentigos can evolve into melanoma, usually slowly, over many years. A benign
lentigo first becomes a lentigo maligna, which is analogous to an atypical
mole. If not removed, the lesion may eventually become a melanoma. The
lentigo maligna melanoma shown here is very large and has marked color variegation and irregular borders; biopsy confirmed it as melanoma. The lesion
above it probably is a benign lentigo or possibly a lentigo maligna; it, too,
should be removed or watched closely for signs of change. By permission of
Anti-Cancer Council of Victoria.

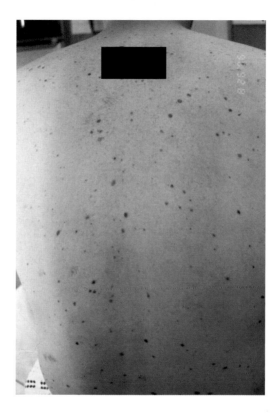

PLATE 13. Person with severe atypical mole syndrome: note multiple large moles, most with atypical features. This person has germline mutations in both copies of the p16 gene. Only in his twenties, he has already had two primary melanomas.

4

Skin Warning Signs

Melanoma can develop in two ways. Most commonly, an existing mole (often present for many years) gradually begins to change and eventually becomes cancerous. Sometimes, however, melanoma develops directly from melanocytes residing at the junction between the dermal and epidermal layers of skin. It appears on the skin as a new mole that never has a stable appearance (as it should) but rather continues to change gradually. The development of melanoma in this way is referred to as *de novo*, literally meaning "anew." Most people do not continue to acquire new moles after the age of 30, so the development of a new nevus later in life may signal the de novo development of melanoma. Such moles should be excised or at least monitored very closely for continued change. In some cases, what appears to be a new mole may actually be a lentigo; lentigos, in contrast to nevi, appear more frequently as we age. They are often impossible to distinguish from moles unless they are removed and examined under a microscope.

The Appearance of a Normal Mole

Because most melanomas probably develop from existing moles, it is very important to be able to recognize the characteristics of a benign or normal mole, as well as the changes in a mole that may suggest it is becoming malignant. A normal mole is round or oval and symmetrical (one half of the mole looks identical or nearly identical to the other half). It is also well defined and even around the edges, so that it is easy to distinguish the mole from the surrounding skin. It may be completely flat, or it may be raised to some degree depending

| *Do most melanomas develop de novo or from existing moles?* | Faced with a case of melanoma, a doctor cannot say with certainty what took place in the months or years before to cause that malignant spot to be where it is. Nonetheless, four pieces of evidence suggest that most melanomas |

develop from existing moles.

First, the more moles a person has, the more likely he or she is to develop melanoma. Second, serial photographs have documented the development of melanoma in existing moles. Third, as many as 85% of patients diagnosed with melanoma remember having a mole, often for many years, at the site of their melanoma. Finally, when *thin* melanomas are examined microscopically, up to 70% of them are seen to contain remnants of a benign mole. This suggests that the mole has undergone malignant changes. (The proliferation of cancer cells in larger melanomas would obliterate any evidence of a benign mole.)

on whether it is a junctional, compound, or intradermal nevus (see Chapter 2). Most normal moles range between 2 and 6 millimeters (less than a tenth of an inch to nearly a quarter of an inch) in diameter, though some are larger. Finally, the color of a benign mole is uniform throughout. It may be the same color as the person's skin or any shade of brown, from tan to nearly black.

Most individuals have moles that are similar in size and color. One person may have small moles that are light in color while another has larger, darker moles. The color tends to be lighter in people with fair skin and darker in people with naturally dark skin. Like skin color, mole color is related to the type of melanin the person produces.

New moles arise normally only until a person is around age 30. Often more than one will appear at the same time. They usually appear in sites that have previously received significant sun exposure.

WHAT TO WATCH FOR

In Chapter 2, we described the natural slow and gradual evolution of a new mole from a junctional mole to a compound mole to an intradermal mole, until it finally disappears. These changes occur over decades, and they are so gradual that they are seldom noticed. Once a mole has fully developed, it should appear to be the same size, shape, and color for many years. In addition, a normal mole will never bleed, itch, burn, or hurt unless you accidentally knock or scrape it or you have an overlying skin rash or condition, such as eczema, psoriasis, or shingles.

Several years ago, the American Academy of Dermatology developed a set of melanoma warning signs or changes in a mole that may herald the development of melanoma. These warning signs—**a**symmetry, irregular **b**orders, **c**olor variegation, and large **di**ameter—have been called the **ABCD criteria** and are described in Plate 8. We will discuss them in more detail below.

Unfortunately, once all of the classic ABCD features are present in a lesion, it is likely that invasive melanoma has already developed. Because melanoma proceeds through a recognizable precancerous stage, the goal should be to identify it *before* it has advanced to the cancerous form. Removal of the lesion at the precancerous stage will prevent the potentially lethal form from developing.

The premalignant lesion from which most melanomas arise is called an **atypical** or **dysplastic nevus.** Both terms are commonly used, and we will use them interchangeably. An atypical nevus is part of the continuum in the development of melanoma from a normal melanocyte to invasive melanoma. Fortunately, just as all moles do not become atypical, not all atypical moles will go on to become melanoma. This is because progression to melanoma requires further "hits" or damage to the genes that regulate melanocyte growth. As many as 5–10% of Caucasian adults have at least one atypical nevus, but only 1–2% of Caucasians develop melanoma. Unfortunately, we currently have no way of knowing which atypical nevi will go on to become melanoma and which will not.

Atypical nevi are located along the continuum between normal moles and melanoma, so it is not surprising that atypical nevi both on the skin and under the microscope *look* like they fall somewhere between the two (see Plate 9, *A–D*). Like melanoma, dysplastic moles usually develop either from junctional nevi or from the junctional component of compound nevi. The smaller the junctional component of a nevus, the less likely it is to transform into melanoma. Therefore, the moles you should monitor most closely for change are those that are either completely flat or have a flat component. Unfortunately,

| *Atypical nevi under the microscope* | Strictly speaking, atypical, or dysplastic, nevi are moles with abnormal microscopic features. Two types of abnormality may be seen under the microscope: architec- |

tural disorder and cytologic atypia. *Architectural disorder* refers to an irregular pattern of growth of the melanocytes composing the mole. This pattern is clearly different from the well-defined clumps of melanocytes or nevus cells that compose benign moles, but it is less extreme than the wildly disordered pattern that characterizes the growth of invasive melanoma cells.

Cytologic atypia refers to cellular changes in the melanocytes composing an atypical mole. These changes might include an increase in the size of the nucleus, changes in the size or shape of the melanocytes, or evidence that the melanocytes are dividing. Again, these changes are abnormal but are less severe and less prevalent than those in actual melanoma cells.

Atypical nevi are graded according to the severity of the microscopic changes that are seen. The pathologist will describe them from the least to the most severely abnormal as follows:

- nevus with architectural disorder,
- nevus with architectural disorder and mild cytologic atypia,
- nevus with architectural disorder and moderate cytologic atypia,
- nevus with architectural disorder and severe cytologic atypia.

The next steps are melanoma in situ and, lastly, invasive melanoma.

however, mole subtype cannot always be determined by the naked eye. A mole that appears to be completely raised (intradermal), may on examination under a microscope prove to have a flat (junctional) component. So, although you should pay most attention to flat or partially flat moles, changes in raised moles should not be ignored.

Although all the ABCD features in a skin lesion—asymmetry, irregular borders, color variegation, and large diameter—are usually seen with invasive melanoma, the appearance of only one or two of these signs may be seen in an atypical nevus. For example, color variation in a small, symmetrical mole with well-defined borders may be a sign that the mole has become dysplastic. In addition, the changes that mark the development of an atypical nevus are usually more sub-tle than those that signal melanoma. A dysplastic nevus, for instance, may show an egg-shaped *asymmetry* in which one-half of the mole does not match the other, but this asymmetry is usually not nearly as marked as that of a typical invasive melanoma. The *borders* of an atyp-ical mole are often seen to blend into the surrounding skin or to be mildly irregular, but the irregularity is usually much less extreme than the prominent notching that is often seen in the borders of an invasive melanoma.

Color variegation is one of the most common changes seen in atypical nevi. Different shades of brown or pink blotch these moles rather than the deep blue, red, or white colors that may appear in melanomas. A distinctive deep blue, almost black, color results when large amounts of melanin are present deep in the dermis. This occurs in invasive melanoma but not in dysplastic nevi. Red is a sign of **in-flammation,** which frequently occurs in melanoma but, again, is gen-erally not a feature of atypical moles. A white color (an area where pigment is lost) results when the immune system reacts against and destroys melanocytes. This, too, generally does not occur in dysplas-tic moles but frequently occurs once melanoma has developed. (Im-mune attack against melanocytes may also occur in the benign condi-tion known as **vitiligo,** but this tends to result in large patches of unpigmented skin rather than in a pigmented lesion with one or more white regions.) A whitish color sometimes appears surrounding, but not within, normal or atypical moles. When this occurs, the nevus is referred to as a **halo nevus.** Halo nevi may be solitary or multiple and may be associated with vitiligo. Their significance is not known.

Diameter is the least useful of the ABCD criteria. In fact, many specialists think it should be dropped altogether. The diameter crite-rion states that we should be concerned about pigmented lesions larger than 6 millimeters (about a quarter of an inch) in diameter. This standard was initially developed because normal moles are usually small, dysplastic moles are often larger, and melanomas are frequently larger yet—often more than 1 centimeter (about half an inch) across. Atypical nevi and melanomas both may be smaller than 6 millimeters in diameter, however, and if the ABCD criteria were strictly adhered to, these lesions would pass the test of normalcy. Plate 10 shows a mole with all four ABCD criteria.

A benign nevus should remain stable in size, shape, and color for many years. Any change in a pigmented lesion should always raise a big warning flag that the nevus may be changing into melanoma. It may be a change in size, shape, color, symmetry, or surface contour, or it may be the development of itching, tingling, burning, bleeding, crusting, or scaling, with or without a change in size, shape, or color. Changes that are causes for concern generally occur over a period of weeks to months. Changes that take place over a few days and then subside are usually the result of local inflammation or injury rather than the development of melanoma. One caveat: changes in skin color and mole color may occur naturally during pregnancy and do not necessarily signify the development of melanoma, but any changing moles must be monitored carefully, even during pregnancy (see Chapter 12).

AMELANOTIC MELANOMA

Amelanotic melanoma is melanoma in which the melanoma cells do not make melanin. As you can probably guess, these melanomas are not pigmented, although they may appear pink or red (see Plate 11). Because the skin lesions are not pigmented, patients and physicians alike seldom consider the possibility that they may be melanoma. Instead, they are usually assumed to be some benign condition such as a pimple, a bug bite, or a minor infection. Because melanoma can be amelanotic, you should be suspicious of any skin lesion—pigmented or not—that meets any of the criteria discussed above, and seek medical attention if the lesion persists for longer than 4 weeks.

Dawn's Story

Dawn, a 47-year-old homemaker from Australia, describes her experience with amelanotic melanoma: "In July 1995, I developed the flu and visited my doctor. During that visit, I also pointed out a small mark on the side of my nose that was not unlike a small pimple or bug bite, but it had been present nearly three months. I was told this was only an infection under the skin and was prescribed antibiotics for the flu and was told the antibiotic pills would also help the infection on my nose. I was still feeling poorly with the flu in August and returned to the doctor's office. I again mentioned the mark on my nose, but my doctor was not concerned. By Christmas time, I was becoming quite concerned about the pimple, which persisted and was becoming larger. I returned to my doctor to request a referral to a local surgeon. The surgeon removed the mark. I still recall vividly the moment my husband and I were called into his office a few days later to be told that the spot on my nose was a rare form of melanoma, called amelanotic melanoma. It is hard to describe how we felt."

Doctors can now find no trace of melanoma elsewhere in Dawn. But to prevent its spread, Dawn underwent three additional operations.

In addition to the ABCD criteria, change in any pigmented (or unpigmented) lesion, and the appearance of a *new* mole on a person over age 30, there is one other warning sign that should cause concern. Any mole that is *out of character*, or different in appearance, from a person's other moles should be considered suspicious and probably removed. For example, if a fair-skinned person with lightly colored nevi notes a single darker nevus, he or she should consult a physician about it, even though it may be lighter than all of the moles of a darker-skinned friend.

There are always reasons not to check your moles regularly or not to consult your doctor when they appear to be changing. We all lead busy lives, and a mark on your skin may seem inconsequential.

---

*F*eatures of skin lesions that should concern you

- A nevus with any of the ABCD criteria
- Any change in a nevus, including bleeding, scaling, crusting, pain, or change in size, shape, color, symmetry, or surface contour
- Any new nevus developing after age 30
- Any nevus that is out of character for you—for example, one that is significantly darker or larger than your other moles

The results of neglect can be devastating, however. The importance of monitoring skin lesions cannot be overstated.

Jim's Story

Jim was a healthy 34-year-old who worked as a conductor on a commuter railroad. When he wasn't at work, he spent time with his large family and his many friends. He was also active in his church. It seemed that he was always driving someone somewhere or doing an errand to help someone else. When he first noticed the unusual mole on his neck, he didn't pay much attention to it. His wife noticed it too and suggested Jim ask his doctor about it. But Jim had grown up in a family that prided itself on its good health and on its ability to "tough things out." They joked a lot about friends they considered to be hypochondriacs— people who ran to the doctor every time they sneezed.

By the time Jim went for the checkup mandated by his job, the mole had changed a good deal. It was bigger and had turned blue-black in color. The doctor noticed the mole and told Jim that it would have to be removed. Reluctantly, Jim made an appointment for the procedure. The pathologist's report showed that the mole was a Clark's level IV melanoma. Jim had to have a second operation to be sure that all the melanoma cells in the initial site had been removed. He made light of the whole thing when he went back to work, but a year later he developed swollen lymph nodes in his neck near where the melanoma was removed. A needle biopsy proved that Jim's glands were filled with melanoma, and he had to undergo major surgery to remove them.

Jim then took Interferon shots, which made him a bit weak and tired, but he did okay until a year and a half later, when a routine X ray of his lungs showed that the melanoma had spread there. A **CT scan** determined that the melanoma was also present in his liver. Now, four years later, despite several **chemotherapy** treatments, the cancer has spread to Jim's brain, and he can no longer work or participate in the many activities he used to enjoy. He and his family are having to face the fact that he does not have long to live.

PREMALIGNANT LENTIGOS

Because lentigos, like moles, are caused by an increase in the number of melanocytes, they too can undergo transformation into a premalignant form (like the dysplastic nevus) called **lentigo maligna,** or **Hutchinson's melanotic freckle** (see Plate 12), and eventually into a particular subtype of melanoma, known as **lentigo maligna melanoma** (see Chapter 7). For this reason, we need to watch lentigos for the warning signs described above in the same way we monitor nevi. The only important difference between the two is that, for reasons we do not yet understand, the malignant transformation of a lentigo, or lentigo maligna, usually takes place more slowly than it does in a nevus or an atypical nevus.

WHO CAN HELP MONITOR MOLES?

The unfortunate situation is that many physicians are poorly trained in recognizing the warning signs of melanoma. Melanoma has become a major health concern so rapidly that medical training has not kept pace. Currently in the United States, most medical students, interns, and residents not specializing in dermatology receive little, if any, education about the need to screen for melanoma and its precursor lesions, let alone about which pigmented lesions they should watch most carefully. In addition, most people visit their doctors only when they are sick or injured or for annual checkups, where they are examined for a wide variety of health markers that are more routine. Both patient and doctor often focus on symptoms that appear to be of more immediate concern.

You may need to schedule a separate appointment to have an experienced doctor (usually a dermatologist) look carefully at all the moles and other lesions on your skin. Certainly, if you do have moles that show any signs of being atypical or if you remain concerned about any lesion, you should schedule an appointment with a dermatologist. One of the most important points we hope to make in this book is that if you or someone you know has a mole you are concerned about *for any reason*, it should be removed regardless of its appearance. If a physician tells you that a mole you are concerned about "looks fine and is nothing to worry about," ask for a good explanation. Unless you get a good explanation (for example, the lesion may be a classic seborrheic keratosis, which does not involve the melanocytes and can almost always be diagnosed without a biopsy), you should either request that the mole be removed anyway or consult another doctor.

Virtually every expert in pigmented lesions has been surprised when a lesion that looks completely benign and is only removed because of a patient's complaint is found to be a melanoma precursor or even melanoma. Furthermore, it is all too common to find that patients with melanoma had showed the lesion to a physician one or more times in the months or even years prior to being diagnosed with the disease and had been told that it "looked fine" and did not need to be removed. The goal is to remove a lesion *before* it becomes invasive melanoma, not to wait until it is obviously melanoma.

As you will see in Chapter 7, the process of removing a pigmented lesion is simple and carries essentially no risk; thus, little harm is done if a benign lesion is removed. By contrast, the stakes of missing a lesion that is an early melanoma or is changing into melanoma are high. Unfortunately, some people have so many atypical nevi that removing all of them is not practical. Good management of this atypical or dysplastic mole syndrome will be discussed in the next chapter.

Tom's Story

Tom, a middle-aged Caucasian man, had received his medical care for many years at a highly respected hospital in the United States. His major medical problem was a heart condition, which first his primary care physician and then a heart specialist monitored carefully. Sometime in 1993, Tom noticed that a mole just below his left breast seemed to be getting larger, and during his next check-up, he asked his doctor about it. The doctor told him that it was nothing to worry about, and, reassured, Tom paid no further attention to it. In 1995, Tom was admitted to the hospital because of his heart. One of the doctors who cared for him in the hospital happened to have a particular interest in melanoma. The lesion on Tom's chest disturbed her, and she had it removed

Is a mole more likely to turn into melanoma if it is in a place where clothes will rub against it, like on my waist-line?

There is no evidence that this increases the danger of the mole becoming cancerous. Melanoma is, however, much more likely than a mole to bleed with minor irritation. This often prompts the individual to seek medical attention about a lesion he or she might not otherwise have noticed for many more months.

Is it dangerous if I accidentally scrape or cut a mole or get poison ivy on a part of my body where there are moles?

There is no reason to become alarmed if you scrape or cut a mole, but if a mole bleeds or becomes inflamed easily and for little reason, it may be a cause for concern, and it should be excised. Skin rashes such as poison ivy are not related to the development of melanoma.

the next morning. The biopsy results indicated that it was an invasive malignant melanoma. (Plate 9*D* is a photograph of Tom's melanoma.)

Over the two years between the time Tom first mentioned the mole to his doctor and his admission to the hospital, several very good doctors had laid their stethoscopes over the lesion while listening to his heart. None of them, apparently, recognized the potentially dangerous nature of the lesion.

...

5

What Is Your Risk?
The Risk Factors for Melanoma

We know that melanoma is associated with sun exposure, but we also know that some people are more likely than others to develop melanoma, even when they have the same amount of exposure to the sun. By comparing large groups of people who have or have not contracted melanoma, physicians have discovered a number of personal characteristics that are associated with it. These characteristics are known as **risk factors.** Being familiar with these risk factors is extremely important.

People at high risk for melanoma need to be especially careful to implement preventive measures. They and their doctors must also be vigilant in looking for changes that may signal the onset of melanoma, so that any occurrence of the disease can be detected as early as possible. In this chapter, we will discuss the most important risk factors for the development of melanoma. We will start with the risk factors that are shared by much of the Caucasian population and then will spend some time on the **atypical mole syndrome,** which affects a small percentage of the population but is the greatest risk factor for the development of melanoma. Using the worksheet at the end of the chapter, you can estimate your own personal risk for developing the disease.

CHANGING MOLES

We devoted all of Chapter 4 to describing changes in a mole that may herald the development of melanoma. A mole that is changing in any way is of concern and should always be evaluated by a professional.

Number of Moles

As we mentioned in Chapter 3, the more moles you have, the greater your risk for developing melanoma. This is true even if none of your moles have atypical or precancerous features. This is really not surprising, since most melanomas seem to develop from moles.

The number of moles a person has is determined by a combination of factors, but the two most important are probably genetics and sun exposure. Researchers have found that identical twins (who have identical genes) usually have similar numbers of moles. Fraternal twins or other siblings (who share only some of their genes) are less likely to resemble each other in this respect, just as they are less likely to have the same hair color or eye color.

There is also little doubt that number of moles is related to sun exposure. As we noted in Chapter 3, moles (and melanomas) are most common on parts of the body that receive the most intense, intermittent sun. Caucasians living in tropical and subtropical climates have more moles than those residing in temperate climates.

There is also some evidence that the immune system plays a role in determining the number of moles a person has. People infected with the AIDS virus, people who have had organ transplants, and people who have been on medications that suppress the immune system tend to have more moles.

Atypical Moles

Atypical moles may serve as precursors to melanoma, and they also serve as a general marker of people at risk for melanoma. As with benign moles, the more you have, the greater your risk. As many as 5–10% of Caucasians will develop at least one atypical mole in their lifetime, but most of these people do not have atypical mole syndrome. So as long as these atypical moles are removed or closely monitored for change, the increase in their risk is not that great.

Congenital Moles

We discussed congenital moles in Chapter 2. Those that are less than 2 centimeters (about three-quarters of an inch) across are probably not at greater risk of becoming melanomas than moles acquired after birth, but those that are larger do pose a greater risk, and the risk increases with the size of the mole. The very large form known as giant congenital nevi have a 5–10% lifetime risk of developing into melanomas, and half of these melanomas develop in the childhood years.

INTENSE, INTERMITTENT SUN EXPOSURE

Surprisingly, outdoor workers have not been shown to be at high risk for developing melanoma. By contrast, people with a high educational and socioeconomic status who have indoor occupations have been. In addition, melanoma is most common on body parts most likely to receive intense, intermittent sun—the back in men and the legs in women (each location accounts for 40% of all melanomas in the respective sexes)—rather than the head, neck, hands, and forearms, areas that receive regular sun exposure.

These observations and others have led researchers to conclude that intense, intermittent sun exposure is a bigger risk factor for melanoma than chronic, steady sun exposure. For example, a lawyer who works indoors 12 hours daily, six days per week, sees very little sun all week. But then, to release stress, he goes for a 4-hour bike ride on Sunday from 10 A.M. to 2 P.M.—the peak hours of UV exposure (see Figure 6.1). That same lawyer is also likely to have the financial resources to take frequent vacations in the tropics. Doctors and scientists now believe that repeated episodes of intermittent, intense sun exposure are a real risk factor for melanoma and should be avoided, particularly by people with other risk factors. Sun exposure can be significantly reduced without compromising lifestyle by regularly implementing the protective measures discussed in Chapter 6.

PRIOR SEVERE SUNBURNS

Sunburn is the ultimate evidence of intense, intermittent sun exposure, and almost every epidemiological study ever done on melanoma has shown that a history of severe sunburns in childhood is associated with an increased risk of melanoma. The more times you have been sunburned, the greater the likelihood that you have set the stage for melanoma to develop. Each sunburn causes major damage to the DNA of the skin cells, and the damage accumulates with each burn, since melanocytes last a lifetime.

The ill effects of sunburn—which include wrinkles, lots of ugly spots, and nonmelanoma skin cancer, in addition to melanoma—usually do not show up for many years. There is therefore no immediate incentive (other than the discomfort of the sunburn) for young people to discontinue their bad sun habits. By the time they are adults, they will probably experience far less sun exposure, but unfortunately the damage has already been done. This is why we urge everyone to teach their children good sun habits early.

MELANOMA IN A CLOSE RELATIVE

Most people diagnosed with melanoma do not have a family history of the problem. Ten percent of patients, however, do have one or more first-degree relatives with the disease (your first-degree relatives are your parents, your brothers and sisters, and your children). Most of this is not due to a true inheritance of the disease but, rather, to the fact that we often inherit the same skin type and tendency to form moles as our parents; we frequently have had similar amounts of sun exposure as our parents, as well.

By contrast, as we explained in Chapter 3, in rare cases melanoma actually can be inherited. In other words, certain genes that predispose a person to melanoma may be passed on from generation to generation. These inherited gene abnormalities (germline mutations) are relatively uncommon and are usually brought to light when a *number* of family members over several generations suffer from the disease. For most people the risk associated with having a single first-degree relative who has been diagnosed with melanoma ranges from 2 to 12 times the average risk of getting the disease. For people from a "melanoma family," however, the risk is as high as 100%.

Because of the potential risk, you should get to know your family's medical history and should let family members know if you are diagnosed with melanoma so that they can take appropriate preventive measures.

PERSONAL HISTORY OF MELANOMA

People who have had one melanoma are at greater-than-average risk for developing additional primary melanomas. For most melanoma patients this risk is about 1–5%, but for people with the atypical mole syndrome the risk is much higher. All melanoma patients should take extra care in getting to know their remaining moles and examining them regularly. They should also have full skin examinations at regular intervals (at least every 6 months), with removal of any worrisome lesions. Fortunately, most melanoma patients are vigilant and know what signs to look for, so most of these subsequent melanomas are discovered early and removed before they become dangerous.

SKIN TYPE

A common characteristic of melanoma patients is fair skin. Indeed, the likelihood of developing melanoma is directly related to skin color—the lighter your skin, the greater your risk. That being said, however, there are still many Caucasians with skin that tans easily who develop melanoma. Even people with naturally dark skin, such as Africans and Indians, occasionally get the disease, though this is uncommon.

HAIR COLOR

There is a common misconception that most people who develop melanoma have red hair, probably because we often associate redheads with fair skin. Although the percentage of melanoma patients who have red hair (12–15% in the United States) is higher than the percentage of redheads in the general population (6–8%), most melanoma patients in the United States have light to medium brown or blonde hair. The percentage of melanoma patients with red hair may be higher in Australia and Britain due to a greater percentage of redheads in their populations.

AGE

Although much of the skin damage that leads to melanoma occurs early in life, when we receive most of our sun exposure, most melanomas do not appear until adulthood. The risk of developing melanoma, like the risk of most cancers, increases with advancing age. In the past, the average age at the time of diagnosis of melanoma was 45, but recent years have seen a decline in age at diagnosis, with many people now developing melanoma in their 20s and 30s. As noted in Chapter 3, melanoma is the most common form of cancer in Australian males aged 25–59 and is second only to breast cancer in females in the same age group. It is also the second most common form of cancer in both males and females aged 15–24. This trend is thought to reflect greater sun exposure earlier in life. Melanoma in children is uncommon but not unheard of (see Chapter 12).

GENDER

There is no evidence that one sex is more prone to melanoma than the other. On average, women who do get the disease have slightly fewer **recurrences** than men. A trend toward increasing incidence in men, particularly in Australia, is probably due to changing lifestyles.

SUPPRESSION OF THE IMMUNE SYSTEM

We have learned only in the last decade that people with a suppressed or weakened immune system seem to be at an increased risk for developing melanoma. Specifically, people who require immunosuppressive treatment after a bone marrow or organ transplant and people infected with the AIDS virus have been shown in scientific studies to have an increased likelihood of developing melanoma. Because weakening of the immune system has only recently been identified as a risk factor for melanoma, few details are known. It is curious, though, as we have already mentioned, that these same people tend to develop more moles. More studies will certainly be done to investigate this risk factor further.

PRIOR PUVA TREATMENTS TO THE SKIN

PUVA (an abbreviation for "psoralen and ultraviolet A") is a specialized type of ultraviolet light therapy used to treat severe forms of the skin disorder psoriasis. Not surprisingly, patients who have received prolonged PUVA therapy (more than 250 treatments) have more than five times the average risk of developing melanoma. Most of these melanomas occur 15 or more years after the PUVA treatments began.

XERODERMA PIGMENTOSA

Xeroderma pigmentosa is an extremely rare condition, but you may have heard about it because it is associated with an extremely high risk of developing both melanoma and nonmelanoma skin cancers. This is because affected persons have a defect in what are called *DNA repair enzymes.* These enzymes are the tools used by cells to repair the everyday damage that occurs to our DNA. Without these very important enzymes, skin cells have no hope against the sun's potent UV rays.

ATYPICAL MOLE SYNDROME

The strongest risk factor for the development of melanoma is the **atypical mole syndrome,** which is also known as the **dysplastic nevus syndrome.** Only a small percentage of the Caucasian population have this condition (less than 1%), but it is important because of its close association with melanoma. The syndrome was first described by Dr. Wallace Clark (of Clark's levels) and his colleagues in 1978. They reported the frequent presence of unusual moles in many members of six families with hereditary melanoma. These moles tended to predominate on the upper torso and arms. They were large, averaging 1 centimeter (about half an inch) in diameter, and irregular in outline. Their pigmentation had a very haphazard mixture of pink, tan, and various shades of brown, and they frequently could be felt to have a slightly raised component, although they appeared completely flat to the naked eye.

In addition, Dr. Clark and his associates noted a striking variability between the different moles on the same person. Plate 13 shows a person with atypical moles very similar to those of the patients in Dr. Clark's initial report. In this report, Dr. Clark and his colleagues dubbed this condition the "B-K mole syndrome" after the initials of two young patients from the original families in the study. Between them, these patients had been diagnosed with seven primary melanomas, despite their young age. In addition to appearing unusual to the naked eye, these moles also had atypical or precancerous features when viewed under the microscope, and serial photographs documented the transformation of two such atypical moles ("B-K moles," as they were then called) into melanoma over time. This provided the first evidence that in addition to serving as a marker of increased melanoma risk, B-K moles might be actual precursors to melanoma.

As if this syndrome didn't already have enough names, you may also hear it referred to as the FAMM syndrome, which stands for **familial atypical mole and melanoma syndrome.** This name is misleading, however, since some persons with the syndrome do not have a family history of melanoma or even a family history of atypical or multiple moles. In fact, there are now considered to be two subtypes of the atypical mole syndrome: familial (or hereditary) and sporadic, in which there do not appear to be other family members with either the atypical mole syndrome or melanoma. Scientists believe that sporadic cases represent a new genetic mutation, rather than one that has been passed on from generation to generation.

Since the initial reports of the atypical mole syndrome, it has become clear that not all people with the syndrome have moles that fit the original B-K mole description. For example, the nevi may be smaller and they may not have the striking variability from mole to mole mentioned in the initial report. There may also be an "inverse pattern," particularly in women, where the majority of nevi may be on the legs rather than on the back, chest, and arms as described by Dr. Clark. Finally, both the total number of moles and the number of atypical moles can vary significantly from person to person. The wide variability in the nevi observed in people with the atypical mole syndrome is probably due to different genetic mutations. This has not been proved, but it has recently been shown that only 15% of persons with a history of multiple primary melanomas (many of whom have the atypical mole syndrome) have inherited an abnormal p16 gene. The assumption is that the other 85% have different genetic mutations that have not yet been identified, and that each different mutation may express itself in its own distinct way.

Because of the variability of the atypical mole syndrome, it is sometimes difficult to decide whether a patient has the syndrome or not. The most widely accepted criterion is the presence of more than 100 total body moles, at least 10 of which have atypical features when viewed on the skin and/or when examined under a microscope. As you might imagine, the diagnosis is not an exact science. It is difficult to make a precise count of the total number of moles you have or the number with atypical features, especially if you have lots of moles. The experience of the doctor and factors such as a personal or family history of melanoma or atypical nevi play an important role in making a diagnosis. If you feel you may have an abnormal mole syndrome, you should be diagnosed by a specialist who has examined hundreds of people with numerous moles.

Although a microscopic examination of your moles is not required for a diagnosis of the atypical mole syndrome, usually one or more of the most abnormal-appearing moles are removed through a very minor surgical office procedure called a **biopsy** (see Chapter 7) for microscopic review. If atypical microscopic features are noted, the diagnosis of the atypical mole syndrome is confirmed, or *biopsy-proven*. As we have mentioned, the microscopic appearance of a mole cannot always be predicted by its appearance on the skin. For example, moles that appear to be very atypical on the skin may appear completely normal when viewed under the microscope. By contrast, a nevus that appears only mildly atypical to the eye may show definite premalignant features when removed and examined under a microscope.

People who have more than 50 total body moles but do not meet the criteria for the atypical mole syndrome are said to have an abnormal mole pattern. Although they do not have the atypical mole syndrome, these people still have a high risk of developing melanoma. It seems that whatever genetic abnormality results in the propensity to form an unusually large number of nevi also results in a propensity to form mutations leading to atypical or premalignant moles, so the two frequently go hand in hand.

Although, as we have said throughout the text, *most* people do not acquire new moles after the age of 30, people with the atypical mole syndrome or an abnormal mole pattern frequently continue to acquire new moles throughout adult life, even into their 60s and 70s.

In addition, they commonly develop moles in places that are rarely, if ever, exposed to the sun: on the scalp, the feet, the buttocks, the groin, and the female breast. The presence in children of moles in these unusual locations, particularly on the scalp, may be the first indication of the atypical mole syndrome. Removal of nevi on the scalp, even if they do not have worrisome features, may be recommended, since they are difficult to monitor for change. Melanomas that arise on the scalp are frequently very deeply invading at the time of diagnosis because they are not readily noticed at an earlier stage.

As we will see in Chapter 13, a focus of current research is determining which moles are atypical or premalignant before their surgical removal and microscopic evaluation. For now, given the limitations of clinical evaluation and the high stakes involved, a good rule of thumb is that persons with 50 or more total body nevi, including moles which have the atypical features described in Chapter 4, should have at least one of their most atypical moles removed and examined microscopically. This is especially important if they have a close relative who has been diagnosed with either melanoma or the atypical mole syndrome. If the atypical mole or moles are microscopically normal, little harm is done, and the person may be reassured (but should still be reevaluated periodically). On the other hand, if microscopic premalignant features are found, close monitoring is warranted. We will discuss this in detail below.

What is your risk of developing melanoma if you have atypical moles? The risk ranges widely, from as low as 7 times normal to as high as 500 times normal. (In 1996 the "normal" lifetime risk in U.S. Caucasians was 1 in 87. The risk is similar in Europeans but higher for Australians—1 in 30 in 1998.)

There are three different risk groups within this broad range. The lowest risk group includes those who have one or more atypical moles but do not meet the criteria for the atypical mole syndrome. This means people with fewer than 100 total body moles and fewer than ten with atypical features. (Within this subgroup, those with the fewest total moles and the fewest atypical moles are at the lowest risk of all.) The middle risk group includes those who do meet the criteria for the atypical mole syndrome but who have never been diagnosed with melanoma and do not have any close relatives with melanoma.

People at highest risk for the development of melanoma are those with the atypical mole syndrome who either have a personal history of one or more prior melanomas and/or have one or more close relatives with melanoma. In fact, it has been estimated that people with the atypical mole syndrome who come from "melanoma kindreds" such as the family described in Chapter 3, or who have at least two close relatives with melanoma, have a 100% chance of developing melanoma themselves by the time they reach age 70 unless they are extremely vigilant, take proper sun precautions, and have suspicious lesions removed immediately. In addition, people with the atypical mole syndrome tend to develop melanoma at young ages (the 20s is not uncommon); if not monitored closely, these people frequently develop multiple invasive melanomas (see Chapter 12).

In Chapter 4, we urged everyone who has any moles with "warning signs" to have them removed. The fear of developing melanoma has prompted many patients with the atypical mole syndrome to ask if all of their moles can be removed so they can just forget about the whole thing. Unfortunately, this is not practical or even possible for three reasons: First, most people with the atypical mole syndrome have so many nevi that removal of all of them would be extremely disfiguring. Second, most people with the atypical mole syndrome continue to form new moles throughout their adult lives. Finally, melanoma can arise de novo without a preexisting mole, so close monitoring would still be needed.

Many patients have also asked if their moles can be removed with a laser. Unfortunately, this is not possible, either. Lasers can be used for some very thin pigmented lesions such as age spots (lentigos), but moles extend deeper into the skin, and the laser would reach only the top of the mole, leaving the bottom part to "grow back." The other problem with using a laser is that microscopic analysis is not possible for lesions that have been burnt off with a laser. All moles that are removed should be reviewed under a microscope by a pathologist to make sure they have no cancerous features. Again, we must deal with the fact that the microscopic appearance of a mole cannot always be predicted by its appearance on the skin.

Thus, the first line of defense for people with the atypical mole syndrome or even an abnormal mole pattern is *close monitoring*.

Most pigmented lesion specialists (usually dermatologists who specialize in pigmented lesions) agree that this is best done with the aid of **whole-body photography.** As the name implies, this procedure involves having photographs taken of the entire body. In addition, closeup shots are taken of moles with atypical features. These photographs then serve as a baseline to help detect—sooner rather than later—moles that are changing and moles that are new. Having this baseline is particularly important for people with the atypical mole syndrome. They have so many moles (many with atypical features) that the subtle changes that often signal the onset of melanoma may go unnoticed until the melanoma is advanced. Without photographs to help, it is very hard for anyone to remember what an individual mole looked like last month, let alone last year. It is virtually impossible when you have hundreds. (See Plate 13.)

Usually two copies of the whole-body photographs are made. One is given to the patient to aid in skin self-examinations; the other is kept in the patient's medical file to aid in physician examinations, which should be done every 3–6 months, depending on your risk (see the worksheet at the end of this chapter). Most patients find that these photographs help them keep track of their moles and provide reassurance. Photographs may also reduce the number of moles a person has to have removed. If a mole with atypical features is noted, but comparison with the baseline photographs shows that it is completely unchanged, it can be safely watched. Melanoma does not develop without some evidence of change, although the change may be subtle; atypical moles are dangerous only if they change. In light of our repeated advice that any mole with any warning sign should be removed, this may sound a bit cavalier. It is important to understand, however, that for many people with the atypical mole syndrome, removal of all atypical moles is not possible, since *most* of their moles may have atypical features both to the eye and under the microscope.

Atypical mole patients followed closely with the aid of whole-body photography only rarely develop invasive melanoma, and the development of a deeply invasive melanoma is extremely uncommon. Unfortunately, whole-body photography is currently performed only in highly specialized pigmented-lesion clinics and the cost ($100–$200) is not covered by most insurance plans, public or private. Most patients with the atypical mole syndrome, however, feel that having the photographs is worth the expense.

If you have the atypical mole syndrome, no one should know your moles better than you do. Some patients feel it is just too hard to keep track of their moles, and they want to leave that job up to their doctors. If you decide to take this approach, you are flirting with danger. Your doctor cannot possibly know your moles as well as you can, and change in any one of your moles may occur at any time. Again, we cannot overemphasize the extreme importance of early detection. With the help of a family member or friend, you should do a complete skin examination at least once a month, but don't ignore your moles completely between times. Take note of them while you are in the shower or getting dressed. Make it a habit. If possible, have a spouse or friend periodically check hard-to-see places such as your back and the back of your thighs. If you are concerned about a mole for any reason between scheduled or routine doctor appointments, call and ask your doctor to examine the mole right away. Don't put it off.

Scheduled physician visits (usually with a dermatologist) are the time for a very thorough look at all of your moles, including those in the scalp, between the toes, and in the genital region. If you have whole-body photographs, atypical moles should be compared with them. If you have any questions or concerns, be sure to discuss them with your doctor at this time (making a list before your appointment helps). You and your doctor should then decide which moles, if any, should be removed and checked microscopically. People with the atypical mole syndrome who have had a prior melanoma should also have a physician evaluate them for evidence of recurrence. The timing of these evaluations depends on how long ago your melanoma was diagnosed and what stage it has reached (see Chapter 8). This visit may be with an **oncologist,** a surgeon, an internist, or a dermatologist.

Women with the atypical mole syndrome who become pregnant should pay particularly close attention to their moles throughout their pregnancy, because moles may be stimulated by the hormone surges that occur during pregnancy (see Chapters 6 and 12). In addition to regular skin examinations, people with the atypical mole syndrome should have a yearly examination by an **ophthalmologist** to look for moles in the back of the eye. An ophthalmologist is a physician (an M.D.) who specializes in the eye. It is important that you see a physician for this examination, which requires that your eyes be dilated with special drops.

Because of the high stakes of missing a lesion that may be changing into melanoma and the difficulty people with the atypical mole syndrome face in keeping track of all their moles, we reiterate the policy we advocate for any mole that concerns you: "When in doubt, take it out." Many patients with the atypical mole syndrome have dozens of moles removed over their lifetimes, even those who have whole-body photographs to check against. Most of these people find their many small scars a trivial price to pay to avoid the big scar and emotional distress associated with a diagnosis of melanoma.

Because the atypical mole syndrome is often hereditary and melanoma that runs in families may occur in people with the atypical mole syndrome, all close relatives of people with the atypical mole syndrome should be examined by a specialist at least once. Those with an abnormal mole pattern should be followed closely. Those with a normal mole pattern need not be followed regularly unless they are part of a family in which several members have had a melanoma. In such families, melanoma does develop in members with normal mole patterns, so we recommend that all **first-degree** family members be checked by a physician once a year.

Children of a parent with the atypical mole syndrome should also be evaluated, regardless of whether there is a family history of melanoma. The laws of genetics predict that if one parent has the syndrome (even if it is sporadic), 50% of that person's children will inherit it. These children should have their first examination before they reach puberty. Most children have few moles before puberty, and the development of several seemingly normal moles when a child is between the ages of 5 and 8 may be an early clue that she or he has inherited the syndrome. Another early clue suggesting that a child may be destined to develop the atypical mole syndrome is the presence of moles in unusual locations, particularly on the scalp. The children should be evaluated again in their early teens. Atypical or premalignant changes in moles usually do not appear until the teenage years, and that is also the time when the number of moles may dramatically increase. The goal is to detect the syndrome as early as possible so that strict sun protection measures and frequent skin examinations can be implemented early.

Estimating your risk of developing melanoma

In the following table the **relative risk** number associated with each of the risk factors for melanoma allows you to determine how much more likely a person with a given characteristic is to get melanoma than the general population. Relative risk defines *how much* a risk factor influences the chance of developing a disease by comparing the incidence of the disease in persons with and without the risk factor. Thus, a person with a history of three blistering sunburns is 3.8 times more likely to get melanoma than the general population. A relative risk of 1 is equal to the average risk for the population at large, while a risk of less than 1 reflects a lower-than-average risk. In the table, risk factors are listed in order of highest to lowest relative risk.

If you have more than one of these characteristics, you can determine your risk by multiplying the relative risk numbers associated with each. For example, if you have a total of 50–99 moles (relative risk = 3) and 3 moles with atypical features (relative risk = 7.3) and no other risk factors, your overall risk of developing melanoma is 3 × 7.3 = 21.3 times that of the average person in the population.

Note: These relative risk numbers provide only the *statistical* likelihood of your developing melanoma. A person with few or no risk factors can still get the disease, and a person with a predicted high risk may never get the disease. The relative risk may also be reduced by implementing strict preventive and surveillance measures.

ESTIMATING YOUR RISK OF DEVELOPING MELANOMA

Risk factor	Relative risk*
1. Changing mole	Very high
2. Atypical mole syndrome with two or more first-degree relatives (parents, siblings, or children) with melanoma	500 (100% risk by age 70)
3. Atypical mole syndrome without a personal or family history of melanoma	90–150
4. Xeroderma pigmentosa (rare skin disorder in which skin cells are unable to repair sun-induced DNA damage)	500
5. Giant hairy (congenital) nevus	5–15
6. Personal history of melanoma	9
7. Personal history of nonmelanoma skin cancer	5–15

8. Melanoma in a single first-degree relative (without personal or family history of atypical mole syndrome) 2–12
9. Total body mole number (without atypical moles):
   >100 .... 3.5
   50–99 .... 3.0
   25–49 .... 1.8
   15–24 .... 1.0
   Few or none 0.3
10. Atypical moles:
    1 .... 2.3
    2–4 .... 7.3
    >10 .... ≧12
11. Immunosuppression (in persons, e.g., with organ or bone marrow transplant, AIDS virus infection) 4–8
12. Multiple (>250) PUVA (ultraviolet light) treatments for psoriasis 5.4
13. Red or blond hair 2–3
14. Fair skin that burns easily 2–3
15. Tendency to freckle:
    Mild 1.5
    Moderate to severe 3
16. History of blistering sunburns:
    1–2 .... 1.7
    3 .... 3.8
17. Asian, Hispanic, or African race 0.08–0.15
18. Age <15 .... 0.01

*The relative risk numbers in this table have been derived from scientific studies. In some cases, more than one study has been performed with somewhat different results; in such instances, a range of relative risks have been used.

...

6

Prevention, Early Detection, and Education

No cancer is totally preventable. Cells will sometimes mutate and cancer will sometimes develop, no matter how carefully people conduct their lives. But there are two ways we can reduce our risk of some cancers. The first is by decreasing our exposure to known risk factors, such as cigarette smoke or ultraviolet light. The second is by having regularly scheduled screening tests that are able to detect some cancers at a premalignant state. For some cancers, such as leukemia and brain cancer, little is known about the risk factors and there is no currently detectable premalignant state. Fortunately, for melanoma, we can reduce our risk both by reducing our sun exposure and by monitoring our moles for the warning signs described in Chapter 4. And a mole with warning signs can be excised (cut out) and examined microscopically for signs of cancer (see Chapter 7).

In Chapter 5 we helped you figure out your risk of developing melanoma, but these statistics only give you the odds. Even low-risk individuals sometimes get melanoma. There are some simple preventive measures that you can take to reduce your risk of developing this disease, no matter what risk group you are in. Most people can implement these measures without altering their lives greatly. If you have the atypical mole syndrome or other high-risk factors, you should be especially careful, and you may have to make significant lifestyle changes, but however irritating you may find these measures, they are nothing compared to the anguish of metastatic melanoma.

In the past, much of the emphasis in cancer care has been

on treatment of the disease after it has started. Slowly and steadily, this approach has yielded advances against some cancers. In recent years, however, there has been a gradual shift toward placing greater emphasis on prevention—through education, screening, and earlier diagnosis. Campaigns to reduce tobacco consumption have lowered the incidence of mouth and lung cancers. The widespread use of the Pap smear test has dramatically reduced the number of women dying from cervical cancer. Mammography has meant that many more women have had their breast cancer diagnosed at earlier stages. The result has been less extensive surgery and increased survival rates.

Similar strategies are beginning to take hold in the battle against malignant melanoma. Warnings about the dangers of intense sun exposure appear throughout the United States and Australia before the start of the summer season. Weather reports give UV ratings along with the temperature. Sunscreen sales and use have skyrocketed, and more and more people are asking their physicians to check their moles. As you can see from Figure 3.3, however, the incidence of melanoma continues to grow. This is not because preventive measures do not work, but rather, because people must begin taking preventive measures early in life in order for them to be most effective. Indeed, the incidence of melanoma in the younger age groups in Australia (where educational campaigns were instituted earliest) has begun to decline.

Remember, melanoma isn't the *immediate* result of too much sun. Lie on the beach all day, and all you will notice when you come home is red, painful skin that will probably blister and peel in a not very attractive fashion. Instead, the danger of developing melanoma is long-range and cumulative. Every time you expose your skin to the sun (even if you don't stay out long enough to get burned), you are exposing your melanocytes to UV radiation that may cause them to mutate. If enough of the genes that control cell division are damaged, melanoma may develop. Most adults who do use preventive measures have only been doing so for 5–10 years—well after they have already accumulated most of their lifetime sun exposure (80% of this exposure occurs by age 18). And, of course, the statistics of melanoma incidence include the many people who still take no precautions.

SIMPLE PREVENTIVE MEASURES THAT COULD SAVE YOUR LIFE

Because of the high incidence of melanoma in Australia, the Anti-Cancer Council of Australia initiated an ambitious advertising campaign over 20 years ago to warn people about the dangers of UV radiation and show them how they can protect themselves. Today, this impressive campaign is more active than ever. The campaign's slogan is "Slip, Slop, Slap." This translates into

Slip on a shirt.
Slop on some sunscreen.
Slap on a hat.

It's good advice. Here is some more:

Avoid outdoor activities during the times of highest UV intensity. UV rays are most intense between 10:00 A.M. and 2:00 P.M. standard time (11:00 A.M. to 3:00 P.M. daylight saving time) (see Figure 6.1). In tropic zones they are intense all year long. In temperate zones, they are stronger in summer than in winter. Of course, no one expects you to stay indoors all the time during these hours. Just schedule activities like jogging, swimming, and tennis, that keep you outside for long periods in skimpy clothing, for earlier in the morning or later in the afternoon. When you do go out during these hours—*whenever you go outside in daylight*—do remember to slip on a shirt, slop on some sunscreen, and slap on a hat.

Don't be fooled by cool, hazy days. Remember that you need to protect yourself on days when there is light cloud cover and it is not very hot. UV radiation can penetrate through light clouds, so the outside temperature does not always correlate with UV levels. UV is present in the sun's rays throughout the year, including the winter months, but in varying amounts (less in winter).

Use an effective sunscreen, and use it effectively. Apply sunscreen whenever you are going to be outside in the sun for more than 15 minutes. Apply the sunscreen generously 15–30 minutes before you go outdoors and reapply every 2 hours, no matter what the label says. Have someone else get those spots that you can't reach, and don't forget your feet, ears, and neck. If you are swimming, reapply the sun-

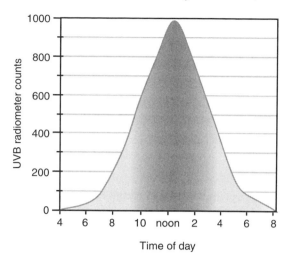

FIGURE 6.1. The intensity of UV radiation at various times of the day. Note that, while UV radiation is present whenever the sun is shining, the intensity is much greater in the middle of the day; these are the times when the sun should be avoided.

screen as soon as you come out of the water, even if the label says the sunscreen is waterproof.

The **SPF** number on the sunscreen is the *solar protective factor*. The higher the number, the greater the protection provided. In general, the solar protective factor indicates how many hours it would take using the sunscreen to get as much UV radiation as you would get with 1 hour of sun exposure without a sunscreen. For example, if the SPF number is 15, you could stay out for 15 hours and get the same amount of UV as if you were out for 1 hour without a sunscreen. For most people, an SPF of 15 is sufficient. You may want to apply zinc oxide cream to highly exposed areas like your nose, ears, and lips. If you are very fair-skinned or have any of the high-risk factors discussed in Chapter 5, you should use a higher number. If you are going to be exposed to very high levels of UV radiation, as you would be skiing at high altitudes or boating, you should also choose a sunscreen with a higher SPF. Water and snow reflect radiation from the sun, making it even stronger. Even dark-skinned people can benefit

Important facts about ultraviolet light

1. UV light reflects off of some surfaces. This can increase the intensity of the rays reaching your skin. Snow reflects the greatest amount of UV light: but sand, concrete, white paint, and water are other culprits. Keep in mind that reflected UV light can reach your skin even while you're under a beach umbrella, and it can reach you under a hat brim. It's best to stay out of the sun completely (that is, indoors) during the peak hours of sunlight.

2. UV levels are significantly higher at high altitudes because the thinner atmosphere of high altitudes filters out much less UV. Remember this when mountain climbing or skiing—and don't forget about the snow's great ability to reflect UV back onto your face or other unprotected areas.

3. UV light can damage your eyes. To prevent the sun from causing cataracts, wear sunglasses that provide UVA/UVB protection. Close-fitting wrap-around glasses are best, because the sun can enter the eyes around the edges of most glasses. Sometimes people think that paying a high price for sunglasses automatically means they are getting better protection, but price does not as a rule correlate with the degree of UV protection. *Check the label.* Ask your optometrist about your prescription glasses; a colorless film that screens out UV can be applied to some lenses inexpensively.

4. In addition to the more common "chemical" sunscreens, "physical" sunscreens are very effective at blocking out UVA and UVB rays. The best known (and dreaded by children) is thick white zinc oxide, but there are now others being introduced in formulations that are not thick and white.

5. Car window glass filters out nearly all UVB and at least half of the UVA. You can still get burned taking a long trip on a sunny day, however.

6. A number of medications make your skin sun-sensitive. Be especially careful if you are taking certain antibiotics (ask your doctor or pharmacist), blood pressure medications, immune suppression medications, and even Retin-A (used to treat acne and to counteract the effects of aging). Always read your drug information sheet, and use strict sun precautions while taking such medications.

7. Pregnancy can make you more susceptible to the effects of the sun. Take care, and take cover.

from using sunscreen, although a sunscreen with an SPF of 5 may offer adequate protection.

Recently there has been a lot of media hype about the possibility that sunscreens are not as effective as we once thought at preventing skin cancers. In fact, some claims have been made that sunscreens *cause* skin cancers. Indeed, recent scientific studies have demonstrated both an increased number of moles and a higher rate of melanoma in people with the greatest sunscreen use. Most experts think that the explanation for these findings is that when people use sunscreens, they tend to stay out in the sun for much longer periods of time than they would have without a sunscreen and thus accumulate the same amount of sun damage.

As mentioned in Chapter 3, both UVA and UVB rays cause cancer and aging of the skin, while UVB rays cause most of the effect of sunburn. Until recently, most sunscreens provided only UVB protection—preventing sunburn but not preventing penetration of the UVA rays of the sun. While we strongly encourage people only to use UVA/UVB sunscreens (these are clearly labeled on the containers), until more studies are available, we do not encourage the use of *any* sunscreen as an excuse to ignore other sun protection guidelines. Sunscreen is not a coat of armor. Again, we strongly advocate its use, *but in combination with other preventive measures* (such as avoiding the hours of peak sunlight) to protect your skin from the damaging effects of the sun that can lead to melanoma. We do not have specific recommendations about particular brands of sunscreens. Read the labels and find one that is right for you and your skin.

Wear protective clothing. Clothing that covers your skin—long-sleeved shirts with collars and long pants, especially those made with densely woven material that you can't see through—give the best protection from the sun. "Ugh," you say. "Too hot." Maybe not. Even if it is made of sturdier material, loose-fitting clothing that allows air to circulate is cooler than tight-fitting clothing. And for those with no special risk for melanoma, even lightweight cover-ups may offer sufficient protection. Don't forget to add a hat with a broad brim to shade your face and dark glasses to protect your eyes.

A few companies specializing in sun-protective gear now produce a very lightweight fabric that is UV-resistant. These companies also manufacture a variety of "sun-smart" gear, including special hats

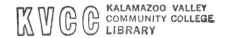

with broad brims and special swimsuits for children (both boys and girls) that cover part of the legs and arms as well as the entire chest, back, and abdomen. These are very popular and readily available in Australia, but unfortunately, thus far they have been less popular and less available in other countries. (See the Guide to Resources at the end of this book for information about how to buy this gear.)

Sit in the shade. It is lovely to sit outside in summer. But it is just as lovely to sit under a tree or umbrella that shades you from the sun. A beach umbrella is a good investment, whether you use it by the seaside or in your back yard.

Avoid suntanning salons. Called solariums in some countries, suntanning salons claim that their lights give off a safe form of UV radiation, UVA radiation, which results in a tan but avoids the skin-burning effects of UVB radiation. Surprisingly, no good research studies have been done to determine whether or not using these salons causes melanoma. We do know, however, that UVA radiation penetrates the upper layers of the skin and causes damage to the lower layers as well, causing the skin to wrinkle and age prematurely. As noted above, evidence is mounting that these rays are also cancer-causing. Our advice is to avoid tanning salons unless definitive data eventually prove their safety (an outcome that is unlikely).

Consider the sun when you plan your vacation. Even if you want to vacation by the ocean, choose a spot where there is plenty to do besides lie on the beach. Enjoy less sun-exposed activities when the sun is most intense and save the beach for later (or earlier). Many people in tropical climates eat their main meal at lunchtime and then take a siesta. This keeps them out of the sun during the period of the day when the sun is most intense.

Save the Children

Because the cause of most skin melanomas appears to be intense sun exposure early in life, it is only logical that we should focus on protecting children and adolescents from the sun and, in particular, keeping them from getting sunburned. It is fairly easy to see to it that babies and small children are protected from the sun, but as children get older and are on their own, the job gets more difficult. Here are some suggestions:

Start right away. If children grow up using sensible sun protection, it is more likely to become a natural part of their lives—something they do from habit.

Splurge a little. Buy sunglasses, hats, and cover-ups that are fun or fashionable—things your kids will like to wear.

Keep the sunscreen handy. Get several bottles or tubes. Keep them where you will see them and use them: on the kitchen table, in the car, with the beach toys, in the boat. If your kids carry backpacks, pop one in there too.

Talk to your children about the importance of protecting themselves from the sun. Telling teenagers about the dangers of skin cancer may not convince them to use sunscreens. It may be more effective to tell them they will get wrinkled and ugly, and will develop all kinds of horrid spots that have to be cut off with sharp instruments. When you see someone with terribly sun-damaged skin (especially on their face) discreetly point out to your teenagers that the sun is to blame.

If your child goes to daycare or summer camp, check with the administrators about sun protection routines. Be sure that activities are sensibly scheduled and that the children are required to use sunscreen and wear protective clothing.

Set a good example. Kids really do do what we do, not what we say.

EARLY DETECTION

Unfortunately, many of us have already overexposed ourselves to the danger of the sun, and the seeds for melanoma may have already been sown. For those of us over age 30, it is not what we did last week that is important but what we did all those years ago lying in the sun with just a bikini and baby oil. A refrain in every melanoma clinic from the 35-year-old just diagnosed with the disease is "I haven't sun-tanned for years and I wear sunscreen all the time." Unfortunately, this person didn't behave this way 20 years ago. For those who have had the exposure, early detection and removal of potentially dangerous pigmented spots is the best answer. We do still encourage sun-protective measures later in life, however, since they almost certainly provide some decrease in the risk of melanoma and non-melanoma skin cancers.

We have already warned in Chapter 4 about signs that a mole may be changing into melanoma. Here are some practical suggestions that will help protect you and your family.

Get to know your own moles and those of your children and partner. Have a good look at them and review them periodically for any change in size, color, or shape. You may need a mirror or another person to check your back, neck, buttocks, back of the thighs, and scalp. Ask your physician to check any moles that cause you concern. If you are not fully satisfied with your physician's explanation, get another opinion. Do not ignore moles on young children. Melanoma in children is uncommon, but it is not unheard of.

Ask your physician for a full skin examination. Make this a part of your regular physical exam and that of your children. You may need to schedule a physician visit for just this purpose, to allow for a very careful skin examination, especially if you have several other medical issues to discuss during your regular checkups. People at high risk for melanoma (see Chapter 5) should probably see a dermatologist who specializes in nevi. Encourage your family, friends, and co-workers to schedule their own visits, especially if they have a lot of moles, are fair-skinned, or spend a lot of time vacationing in the tropics.

Monitor congenital nevi. If you or your child has a congenital nevus (a mole that has been present since birth), have it checked out by a specialist.

Stuart's Story

Because Stuart was fair-skinned and had a large number of moles, his college physician referred him to a dermatologist. He considered himself a person who shunned sun-tanning, so he was surprised to learn that his sun exposure was actually excessive. He had had a severe sunburn when he was 14 and had played water polo in outdoor pools throughout his college career. When two of five moles he had removed during a routine dermatology check showed high-grade dysplasia (atypia), his doctor informed him, "Your risk of developing melanoma is about 100% without strict surveillance." (Since this warning, his father and brothers have been diagnosed with melanoma.)

Stuart says he is "perhaps a little more deliberate in spending time with my wife and children." They have routine mole checks around the first of each month and keep 30+ sunscreen in both of their cars as well as in several places around the house. Their children have gotten used to getting "greased up" before they play outside. "Statistics," says Stuart, "are designed to apply to populations, not the individual, but they definitely motivate."

EDUCATION

The most effective means of preventing malignant melanoma and other skin cancers is through education about (1) the dangers of sun exposure, particularly early in life, (2) what skin cancers are, (3) how they develop, and (4) when you should be concerned and have a "spot" checked. In Australia, the intense public education campaigns that have gone on over the last 20 years have clearly shown the benefit of this. In Australians under the age of 40 who have had the benefit of these programs since their younger years, the incidence of malignant melanoma has begun to fall for the first time in 50 years.

Here are some suggestions for educating yourself, your children, your family and friends and your community about melanoma and skin cancer.

- Ask your children's school about initiating an educational program about skin cancer.
- Talk to the administrator of your neighborhood schools about requiring children to wear protective clothing during recess times and scheduling outdoor activities during non-peak sun hours.
- Have your service club or workplace invite an expert speaker on melanoma. Most local cancer societies can provide one.
- Plant some shade trees in your back yard, then show them off to the neighborhood and explain why.
- Collect the Cancer Society pamphlets and newspaper articles on melanoma and skin cancer (they usually come out in the spring) and tack them on the bulletin board at work and at home.

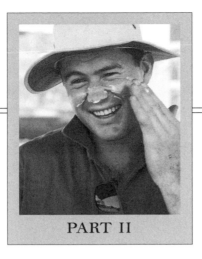

PART II

MELANOMA
Diagnosis and Treatment

Early detection of melanoma decreases the
chances that the cancer will recur or
metastasize to other parts of the body.
A variety of treatments are available for
melanoma. Anyone who has had melanoma
needs to be especially vigilant about
monitoring remaining moles for
any sign of change.

. . .

7

Diagnosing and Treating
the Primary Lesion

I n the first six chapters of this book, we have defined melanoma, described what causes it, and discussed how changes in lifestyle and vigilant examination of moles can help to prevent it. Despite recent efforts to encourage people to protect themselves from the sun and to examine moles regularly to detect any abnormalities or changes, many people (1 in nearly 70 Caucasians in the United States) still develop melanoma. And even if, starting right now, everyone everywhere took careful precautions to avoid melanoma, some people would still develop the disease because of past sunburns and other factors, including genetics. For these people and their relatives and friends, the following four chapters describe how melanoma is diagnosed, what this diagnosis means, and what treatment options are available.

REMOVING THE PRIMARY LESION

The first step in diagnosing melanoma is the suspicion—raised either by a patient or by a physician—that a pigmented lesion on the skin may be melanoma. The lesion from which a diagnosis of malignant melanoma is initially made is called the *primary* lesion. Some experienced clinicians may tell you they can diagnose melanoma simply by looking at a suspicious skin lesion. Certainly, an experienced specialist is more likely to detect the danger signs of melanoma than a doctor who does not commonly examine moles. Strictly speaking, however, *a diagnosis of melanoma can be made only after a lesion has been removed surgically and examined under a microscope.* The process of surgically removing a piece of tissue from any body organ for the purpose of reviewing it microscopically and making a diagnosis is known as a biopsy. The surgery is usually performed by a dermatologist, who will send the excised lesion to a pathologist for analysis.

There are a number of different skin biopsy techniques. The type of biopsy done depends on three factors: (1) the doctor's best estimate of how likely it is that the excised lesion is melanoma, (2) the location of the lesion on the body, and (3) the size of the lesion. If possible, the doctor will remove the entire lesion with a border of normal tissue both around it and underneath it. For lesions less than 1 centimeter (a third of an inch) in diameter, this can usually be done with a procedure called a **punch biopsy.** This technique uses a disposable biopsy tool called a punch. The punch is similar to a round cookie-cutter, but smaller and sharper. Punches come in different sizes. The proper size is one with a diameter slightly bigger than the size of the lesion, allowing a border of normal tissue to be removed around the lesion, while leaving the smallest scar possible.

The doctor performing the punch biopsy will clean the lesion and the surrounding skin to sterilize the area. Then she or he will numb the region with an injection of anesthetic similar to that used by dentists. This injection should be the only painful part of the procedure. The doctor will then place the punch tool over the lesion and rotate it to cut down to the subcutaneous fat. Cutting this deep will almost always leave a border of normal tissue beneath the lesion. The biopsy specimen containing the lesion can then be easily removed. Unless the lesion is very small—less than 2 millimeters (about one-eighth of an inch) in diameter—the doctor will probably close the wound with one or a few stitches to improve healing.

For those lesions smaller than 1 centimeter across, occasionally physicians use a scoop biopsy instead of a punch biopsy, because it will result in a round scar similar to a smallpox vaccination scar, rather than a linear scar that can widen as it heals. In a scoop biopsy, a scalpel is used to make a single scoop-like cut under the lesion. Again, this cut should remove the entire lesion and some surrounding normal skin. Because the wound is more superficial than that made by a punch, sutures are not needed. This technique may have minor advantages, but it requires an experienced hand to be certain the entire lesion is removed and that another procedure is not required.

For larger lesions, the biopsy technique generally used is an elliptical excision, in which a scalpel is used to cut an ellipse around the lesion. This shape allows the edges of a large wound to be brought together without puckering, for a better cosmetic result.

Whatever technique your doctor uses, he or she will protect the wound with a simple dressing, usually just a Band-Aid, and will tell you how to care for it and when sutures (if used) should be removed. The doctor will place the biopsy specimen in a jar with formalin or formaldehyde to preserve the tissue, mark it carefully with your name and identifying number, and send it to the pathology laboratory. The pathologist will embed the specimen in paraffin wax to make it solid. He or she will then cut a number of very thin slices, called *sections*, from the paraffin block, place them on glass slides, and stain them with special dyes so that the fine details of the cells in the tissues become visible. The pathologist will then examine the slides carefully, looking for any malignant or premalignant changes in the cells. This process usually takes 48 to 72 hours.

What the Pathologist Sees

Recall that melanoma develops either from existing nevi that become atypical or, less commonly, from an isolated (non-neval) junctional melanocyte that proceeds along a similar continuum to the development of invasive melanoma. Figures 1.1 and 2.1 show how normal skin and benign nevi appear under the microscope. Normal melanocytes are uniformly spaced along the dermal-epidermal junction, and all appear similar in size and shape. Benign nevi are composed of a cluster of melanocytes, but the melanocytes maintain their usual appearance and their growth is orderly and controlled. In atypical nevi, this orderly growth is lost to some degree ("architectural disorder") and some of the melanocytes may be irregular in appearance ("cytologic atypia"). In melanoma, these architectural and cytologic abnormalities are exaggerated.

Melanoma cells proliferate in a disorderly fashion without regard for neighboring tissues, much as weeds take over a neglected garden. In addition, melanoma cells are not uniform in size or shape. They often contain very large nuclei, and many of the cells may be dividing, a finding that is rarely, if ever, observed in single normal melanocytes or in melanocytes composing a benign nevus. Melanoma cells grow both sideways (radial growth) and downward (vertical growth). The radial growth leads to an increase in the diameter of the malignant mole. It is the vertical growth, however, that allows melanoma cells to gain access to the blood vessels and lymphatics located in the deeper layers of skin. It is these features that the pathologist looks for under the microscope.

Once the pathologist has determined that the cells under the microscope are cancerous, she or he must then determine the melanoma subtype and how deeply it has invaded into the layers of skin below the epidermis. There are four subtypes of melanoma, as defined by their microscopic characteristics:

1. *Superficial spreading:* the most common type of melanoma.

2. *Nodular:* a melanoma that rises above the skin and is often first detected as a lump in the skin, often blue-black in color.

3. *Acral lentiginous:* melanoma arising on areas of the body, such as nailbeds and palms or soles, that do not have hair.

4. *Lentigo maligna melanoma:* a type of melanoma that develops from a lentigo rather than from a mole but is similar in every other way to melanoma arising from a mole.

Doctors used to believe that different melanoma subtypes might have different outcomes—that some might be more dangerous than others. In recent years, however, data have shown that when controlled for depth of invasion, subtype does not influence prognosis. This has led to the present thinking that "melanoma is melanoma is melanoma."

The *depth* to which melanoma cells are found, however, does make a great deal of difference. It is the most important factor in determining how likely the melanoma is to have spread before it was removed. This information provides important guidance for therapy and follow-up. The depth of invasion is determined in two different ways. The first is known as **Breslow's depth.** This technique measures directly in millimeters the distance from the dermal-epidermal

TABLE 7.1. STAGES OF MELANOMA RELATED TO BRESLOW DEPTHS AND
CLARK'S LEVELS

Stage	Breslow depth / metastases	Clark's level
I	0–1.5 millimeters; confined to skin	I, II, III
II	>1.5 millimeters; confined to skin	IV, V
III	Regional lymph nodes involved; no distant metastases; any Breslow depth	Any Clark's level
IV	Distant metastases; any Breslow depth	Any Clark's level

junction to the most deeply invading melanoma cells. The second method is the Clark's level, described in Chapter 3. As with Breslow's depth, the Clark's level for an individual lesion is determined by the level of invasion of the most deeply penetrating melanoma cells. The pathologist's report of a melanoma will usually include the melanoma's subtype and both its Breslow's depth and its Clark's level.

TREATING THE PRIMARY LESION

For many years doctors thought that once they had diagnosed melanoma, the best treatment to prevent its recurrence was to remove all the tissue from a wide area surrounding the primary lesion. This procedure was called a **wide local excision.** The standard until recent years was to surgically excise the normal skin within a 5-centimeter (2-inch) margin of the primary lesion, cutting away all the tissue down to the underlying muscle. This almost always required a skin graft from another site on the body and thus left two large and unsightly scars. Researchers began to question the necessity of such an extensive procedure a number of years ago, and several research studies were carried out to determine if very large excisions really reduced the likelihood that melanoma would recur. These studies showed conclusively that for almost all primary melanomas, smaller, less deforming excisions were just as effective in preventing recurrence. The procedure is still called a wide local excision, but the width of the excision is now determined by the depth of invasion of the melanoma.

In the case of atypical moles that show *severe cytologic atypia,* additional tissue may need to be cut from the margins of the initial excision to be absolutely certain the entire lesion has been removed. With the smaller excisions used today, a skin graft is usually not required. Instead, the wound can be sutured, leaving only a modest scar. Exceptions to this are areas such as the top of the foot and the nose, where the skin is tight and may be difficult to pull together with sutures. In these areas a small skin graft may be needed.

The wide local excision of the primary lesion is usually performed in a physician's office or in an outpatient surgery center. The skin and other tissue removed is sent for pathologic examination to be certain that all of the melanoma has been removed with clear margins. Pathologists use the term **clear margins** to signify that under the microscope a border of normal skin can be seen surrounding every margin of the melanoma tumor. This suggests that all cancerous cells have been removed locally.

By contrast, a pathology report stating that the margins are "positive" means that cancer cells were seen under the microscope right up to the edge of the excised specimen. The presence of **positive margins** strongly suggests that cancer cells have been left behind in the surgical bed. The area should be re-excised surgically when the pathologist reports positive margins. This should ensure that there are no more melanoma cells in the area. Unfortunately, the process is not perfect, and in rare instances melanoma does come back in the region of the primary lesion, even when the margins of the excised tissue were clear. Also, the presence of clear margins does not ensure that malignant cells have not invaded into blood vessels or lymphatic channels present in the skin's dermis or subcutaneous fat before the surgical removal of the lesion. We do not yet have a way of detecting the presence of small numbers of cells that may have spread prior to the initial diagnosis.

QUESTIONS PATIENTS OFTEN ASK

People who have been diagnosed with melanoma are understandably very anxious about their condition, even when the cancer has been caught early and the primary lesion has been surgically removed. The remainder of this chapter deals with some of the questions they often ask.

Will I die from melanoma?

A diagnosis of melanoma is more of an inconvenience than a death sentence for most people. Seventy to eighty percent of all melanoma patients will never have a recurrence or die from the disease. The likelihood that any individual will die of melanoma depends on how far the disease has progressed when it is diagnosed (see Chapter 8).

Would my chances have been better if my melanoma had been discovered earlier?

The longer a melanoma is present before it is removed, the more likely it is to penetrate into the deeper skin layers and spread. On the other hand, most melanomas develop slowly, probably over years, so a delay of a few weeks or even months would not make a difference in most cases.

Should I be cared for by a melanoma specialist or seen in a special clinic?

Anyone with a melanoma invading 1.5 millimeters or more, Clark's level III or greater, and anyone with more than 100 moles should be followed by a physician specializing in melanoma. This may be an **oncologist,** a dermatologist, or a surgeon, depending on which specialty makes you most comfortable. You may choose to be followed at a special melanoma clinic. These clinics are usually associated with large university medical centers and are almost always staffed by a variety of specialists: dermatologists specializing in pigmented lesions, plastic surgeons, medical oncologists, radiation oncologists, specialized cancer surgeons, and pathologists. Support groups are another part of the services generally offered by these clinics. Many patients choose to alternate visits between their primary practitioner and a melanoma clinic, particularly if they live some distance from the specialty clinic; this is an effective means of follow-up as well.

If your primary lesion was less than 1.5 millimeters deep and a Clark's level I or II and you have a normal mole pattern, you can probably receive adequate follow-up from a conscientious general practitioner (although some people still prefer to be followed by a melanoma specialist). Even if you prefer to receive your care from your usual doctor, however, you will probably find that one visit with a specialist is useful. The scientific and medical information about melanoma is changing so rapidly that some general practitioners find it difficult to keep abreast of the latest developments. A visit with a specialist may put to rest some of your fears and may also suggest new diagnostic methods or treatments that should be considered in your case.

Should you or your primary care physician be concerned about any symptoms you have in the future, you will want to be able to consult a specialist you have confidence in. The time of initial diagnosis is a good opportunity to find a specialist you feel comfortable with. The specialist should listen to your concerns and give you clear, frank answers. He or she should accept your wish to obtain a second opinion if you feel it is necessary. The specialist can also provide your doctor with an optimum long-term follow-up plan. The importance of finding follow-up care you are comfortable with is illustrated by Camille's story.

Camille's Story

Camille was 24 years old and eight months pregnant when she noticed a very dark mole on her hip. Because she was so near to term, she decided to wait until the baby was born to have the mole removed. By then, she had noticed two additional moles on her chest that appeared to be changing. When she consulted her primary care doctor, he told her they were nothing to be concerned about, that moles often change during pregnancy. When she insisted that all three moles be removed, her doctor became upset that she did not trust his opinion, but he agreed to refer Camille to a dermatologist. It was an additional three anxious months before she could get an appointment to have the moles removed. The pathology report diagnosed two moles as melanoma and the third as a dysplastic nevus. Since then, Camille has had nearly a hundred moles removed. Three more have been early melanomas, and many more were dysplastic.

Because Camille is so eloquent, we will let her tell the story from here: "Without a doubt, the worst thing about melanoma is the feeling of complete uncertainty of the future. Wondering whether melanoma tumors may be growing inside your body is complete mental torture. When the melanoma was diagnosed, I was referred to a doctor considered exceptional in the treatment of melanoma. With humor, kindness, understanding, and reassurance, he let me know that my multiple melanomas made me 'unusual, but not unique.' And he made me feel for the first time in over a year that I was going to be okay. He helped me realize that every lump, bump, and swollen lymph node was not cancer, took my calls (even though I knew he didn't have time), and fit me into his hectic schedule somehow when I was sure a dizzy spell was a brain tumor. He also was the first doctor who understood that I was not a 'normal' case, that my moles needed to be looked at with a 'different eye,' so to speak. A mole that most people (doctors included) wouldn't think twice about would turn out to be melanoma or at least premelanoma on me. Recently, a researcher tested my blood for defects in the p16 gene, and I tested positive, explaining why I have had so many dysplastic moles and melanomas at such a young age."

If the melanoma does come back, how will I know it? Will it show up as another spot on my skin, or are there other signs or symptoms I should be watching for?

Melanoma is unique among cancers in its ability to spread literally anywhere in the body, but it usually recurs in predictable patterns. The most common place for an initial recurrence of melanoma is in the **lymph nodes** that drain the region of the primary lesion (see Figure 7.1). As you will see in the next chapter, the lymph node basin draining a particular site is often, but not always, predictable.

For example, if a primary melanoma on the left shin spreads to lymph nodes, it will almost always spread first to the lymph nodes in the left groin. A primary lesion located on the middle of the back, however, may spread first to the lymph nodes in either of the armpits, to those in either the groin or collarbone region, or even to either side of the neck. When melanoma spreads to lymph nodes, it shows up as a hard lump or lumps that are usually not painful unless they become very large.

It is important to realize that not all swollen lymph nodes are cancerous. We all get swollen lymph nodes from time to time as a result of infectious or inflammatory processes that we may not even be aware of. People with a history of melanoma are no different. So, if

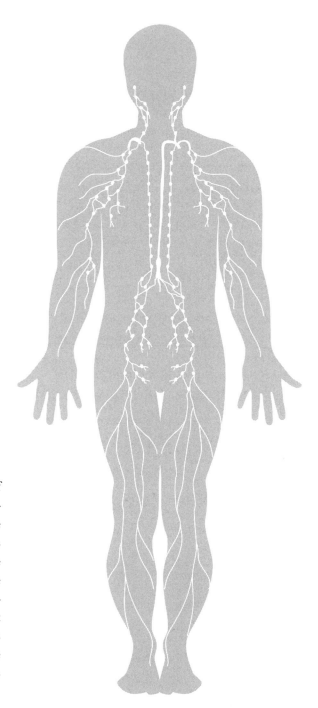

FIGURE 7.1. Distribution of the lymph nodes and the vessels that connect them. Note that there are lymph nodes "draining" most parts of the body. Despite our knowledge of the lymph system, however, we cannot always predict accurately which lymph nodes drain a particular area of the skin without special studies such as lymphoscintigraphy.

you feel a lump you think is a swollen lymph node, don't panic, but do have it evaluated by your doctor.

In other patients, the first sign of melanoma recurrence may be the appearance of a lump or lumps under the skin. These **subcutaneous nodules** may show up either within or near the wide local excision scar or farther away from this site. These are usually very easily seen and felt under the skin, although they are usually not painful. Often they are darkly pigmented (blue or black).

Less commonly, melanoma may spread directly to an internal organ or organs without first showing up in the lymph nodes or under the skin. When it spreads to organs, melanoma most commonly metastasizes to the lungs, liver, and brain, but it may spread anywhere. Melanoma may be present in the internal organs for months or even years before you have any symptoms, because cancer in these locations cannot be seen or felt and usually does not cause problems until the lesions are quite large. Symptoms experienced by people with melanoma that has spread internally vary depending on the organs involved. For example, melanoma in the brain may cause headaches, numbness, weakness, sleepiness, dizziness, or a seizure; melanoma that has spread to the lungs or the heart may cause shortness of breath or cough; and melanoma that has metastasized to the liver or other abdominal organs may cause fatigue or abdominal pain. Other lesions may cause other problems.

We all experience many of these symptoms from time to time, of course. If they are caused by metastatic melanoma, however, they will persist. A headache that is relieved with Tylenol, that is gone in a day or two, or that is typical of a person's usual headaches is almost certainly not the result of melanoma in the brain, nor is a fleeting pain in the abdomen likely to be metastatic melanoma in the liver. You should contact your doctor if you develop any symptom out of the ordinary that persists for more than a few days. Lasting symptoms of any sort may be a sign of some sort of trouble, but not necessarily melanoma.

Lastly, it is important to remember that people who have been diagnosed with melanoma are at an increased risk for developing another primary melanoma (see "Estimating your risk of developing melanoma," p. 62). Therefore, people with a history of melanoma should be especially diligent about monitoring their moles for any of the changes discussed in Chapter 4.

If the melanoma does come back, how soon will it happen? I have heard that for some cancers if you go 5 years without the cancer coming back, you are cured. Is that true for melanoma?

It is true that for some types of cancer, such as cancer of the testicles or uterus, a recurrence is unlikely if it hasn't occurred within 5 years from the time the primary tumor was removed. For melanoma, the average time from removal of the primary lesion to the detection of a recurrence is approximately 4 years, but metastases may occur at any time, from weeks to decades after the initial diagnosis. The longer you go without a recurrence, however, the less likely one is to occur.

Is there a blood test to tell if the melanoma has spread, like the PSA for prostate cancer or the CEA for colon cancer?

No. Currently there is no specific blood test to detect the presence of melanoma cells in the bloodstream, although researchers are working to design such a test. One currently under investigation is called the **tyrosinase test** (see Chapter 13), but for now it is a research tool only. At present, all blood tests used to follow melanoma patients are nonspecific. They merely test your blood for the presence or absence of various components. Elevated or depressed levels of these components can point to problems with various organs, but they do not identify the cause. An increase in the level of a substance called bilirubin, for example, points to liver problems, but there are a multitude of conditions besides melanoma that can cause your liver to function abnormally. Abnormal blood test results are just a signal for further investigation.

Should I have a scan of my whole body to see if the melanoma has spread?

As you will see in the next chapter, this is an area of controversy, but in general it depends on the stage of your melanoma. A negative scan, however, does not mean that the melanoma has not spread.

Will following a special diet, taking certain vitamins, or beginning an exercise program help prevent my melanoma from coming back?

There is no evidence that a specific diet, an exercise program, or some vitamin combination can prevent the recurrence of melanoma. Generally, healthy living with "all things in moderation" is what we advise.

Do I need to stay out of the sun or use special sunscreens?

There is no evidence that further sun exposure increases the risk of recurrence or development of metastases in people with a history of melanoma. Nevertheless, because people who have had one primary melanoma are at risk for the development of a second one, you should take proper precautions in the sun to reduce this risk. These precautions are discussed in detail in Chapter 6. They include avoiding sunburns; wearing protective clothing, sunglasses, and sunscreens; and avoiding outdoor activities when the sun is most intense (10:00 A.M. to 2:00 P.M.). You should be able to implement these measures easily without significantly altering your lifestyle.

I have been under a lot of stress lately. Did the stress cause me to get melanoma?

No one can answer this question with certainty, but no clear link has been established between stress and the development of melanoma. Most of us have some form of stress in our lives, so in retrospect, virtually everyone who gets a serious illness can identify stressful factors that preceded it. Taking reasonable measures to reduce stress is probably a good idea for everyone, if only because it will make life more enjoyable.

What can I do to boost my immune system? Should I be given a cancer vaccine?

What you would really like to do is specifically boost your immune system against melanoma. This is currently being tried using various melanoma vaccines (discussed in detail in Chapters 10 and 13). So far, vaccines are available only as part of experimental trials. Depending on various factors, you might be a candidate for vaccine treatments, but the benefit (if any) of these treatments is as yet unknown. Maintaining or improving your general health by not smoking, getting exercise daily, eating a diet high in fruits and vegetables, and using alcohol only in moderation may generally strengthen your immune system.

Now that I have been diagnosed with melanoma, am I at increased risk for the development of other forms of cancer?

Because many people who develop melanoma have fair skin and a history of sunburns, they are at higher than average risk for the development of nonmelanoma skin cancers—squamous cell and basal cell carcinomas (see Chapter 1). People in melanoma-prone families with mutations in the p16 gene have an increased risk of developing cancer of the pancreas and a particular type of benign brain tumor (meningioma), but these are uncommon. The majority of people with melanoma do not appear to be at any greater risk for the development of other cancers than the general population.

Can I go back to work?

Yes. Once you have recovered from your surgery, there is usually no medical reason why you cannot return to work. Dwelling on the diagnosis of melanoma is common in the first weeks or even months, and different people cope with this differently. For some, returning to a normal lifestyle, including work, helps put things in perspective. For others, a diagnosis of cancer leads to a reassessment of life's priorities and a decision that they want to take more time to "smell the roses."

Now that I have been diagnosed with cancer, can I ever get pregnant?

This is a complicated question, since the health of both the mother and the child have to be taken into consideration. The good news is that in most cases, it is impossible for parents to pass melanoma on to their unborn offspring. Melanoma cells are not carried in sperm, so fathers cannot pass on the disease, even if they are suffering from advanced melanoma. In rare instances, pregnant women with advanced metastatic melanoma pass the cancer on to their unborn children via the placenta, which has numerous blood vessels. This is extremely unusual, however.

Children of people diagnosed with melanoma do have a 2–12 times greater risk of developing the disease than do children without a family history of melanoma. Unless this propensity is due to specific gene mutations, however, it is probably because the children are likely to inherit the same light-colored skin or large numbers of moles that increased the risk of melanoma for their parents. Protection from the sun and observation of moles beginning early in life should significantly reduce this risk. There is no evidence that children with a family history of melanoma are more likely than the general population to develop other types of cancer.

The health consequences of pregnancy for a woman who has been diagnosed with melanoma is a controversial subject, and unfortunately, there are no simple answers. Studies have shown that pregnancy sometimes "stirs up" melanoma cells in women who have been previously diagnosed with the disease. It is not clear why this occurs, but it has led doctors to recommend that women with a history of melanoma delay or avoid pregnancy. Just how long pregnancy should be delayed depends on how deeply the melanoma has penetrated. Your doctor may describe this extent of invasion to you in terms of stages.

We will discuss staging further in the next chapter, but here are the guidelines we believe women should follow: Women who have been diagnosed with melanoma in the upper layers of the skin only (stage I) should delay pregnancy for 2–4 years. Women whose melanoma has been diagnosed as extending into the lower layers of the skin or into the subcutaneous fat (stage II) should delay pregnancy for 3–5 years. Women who have been diagnosed with metastatic melanoma of the lymph glands (stage III) should delay pregnancy 5–10 years. Women with metastatic melanoma that has invaded the organs (stage IV) should not get pregnant.

Women with a history of melanoma should have a thorough examination by a physician to be sure there is no evidence of recurrence of melanoma before they get pregnant. They should also have regular follow-up visits with a melanoma specialist during the pregnancy, in addition to their routine obstetric appointments.

8

Staging, Treatment Decisions, Prognosis, and Follow-Up

In order to determine what kind of treatment is required for any cancer, including melanoma, the doctor needs to determine, as best he or she can, the extent and characteristic of the cancer at the time of diagnosis. This information is necessary for gauging what might happen in the future as well as how often the patient will need to be checked and what tests should be used.

STAGING

Once you have been diagnosed with melanoma, your doctor will probably give you a battery of tests to determine whether or not your cancer has spread from the site of its origin and, if so, to what areas. This series of tests is called **staging.** All the tests in the staging process are aimed at determining whether the cancer is confined to the place it started (*local*); has spread to a nearby area, usually the lymph nodes draining the site of origin (*regional metastasis*); or has spread to internal organs (*systemic metastasis*). At the end of the process, your physician will give your melanoma a stage.

There are four basic stages. As we saw in Chapter 7, in stage I the melanoma is confined to the upper layers of the skin only; in stage II the melanoma has moved into the lower layers of the skin or below the skin; in stage III melanoma cells have spread to the lymph nodes draining the area of the primary lesion; and in stage IV internal organs are involved. The cancer stage determines what treatment and follow-up are appropriate as well as how likely the patient is to have a recurrence of melanoma.

The first step in the staging of melanoma is the pathologist's determination of the Clark's level and the Breslow's depth of invasion of the primary lesion (see Table 7.1). This is followed by a complete physical examination by a physician specializing in melanoma, usually an oncologist. The physical will include a thorough examination of the skin, lymph nodes, lungs, heart, liver, abdomen, and nervous system. Based on the results of the physical exam, the doctor will make an initial diagnosis of the stage of your melanoma. This diagnosis is sometimes referred to as the **clinical stage,** as opposed to the **pathologic stage,** which is based on the biopsy results. Clinical staging is done so that the doctor can decide which, if any, further staging tests to order.

Table 8.1 summarizes the staging system currently recommended for melanoma. If the primary lesion is thin (less than 1.5 millimeters deep), the patient does not have any worrisome symptoms, and the physical examination is normal, no further staging studies are indicated, because the likelihood of finding melanoma elsewhere is extremely small. Other than the sensible follow-up procedures and precautions outlined below, such a patient needs no further testing or treatment at the time of diagnosis. For primary lesions 1.5–4.0 millimeters in depth, a baseline X ray of the lungs, a complete blood count, and blood tests evaluating liver function are recommended. If

TABLE 8.1. STAGING PROCEDURES CURRENTLY RECOMMENDED AT DIAGNOSIS FOR PATIENTS WITHOUT ADDITIONAL SYMPTOMS

Stage	Physical exam[a]	Complete blood count	Liver tests	Chest X ray	Scans	Lympho-scintigraphy or biopsy
I	Yes	No	No	No	No	No
II (less than 4 mm thick)	Yes	No	No	No	No	No
II (more than 4 mm thick)	Yes	Yes	Yes	Yes	Consider	Yes
III	Yes	Yes	Yes	Yes	Yes	Yes
IV	Yes	Yes	Yes	Yes	Yes	No

[a]A complete physical exam for melanoma includes a thorough examination of the skin, lymph nodes, lungs, heart, liver, abdomen, and nervous system. Abnormal findings from this exam or the presence of symptoms may indicate the need for further tests.

these and the physical examination are normal and the patient does not have any symptoms, no further staging studies are usually required. For primary lesions greater than 4.0 millimeters in depth, there is currently no consensus as to how extensive staging studies should be, particularly for patients who have no symptoms or physical examination findings to suggest the melanoma may have spread. We will discuss this further below. Table 8.1 indicates the range of tests your physician may order if he or she thinks they are indicated.

TESTING AND THE LIMITS OF EARLY DIAGNOSIS

Many specialists would argue that no further testing beyond that recommended for patients with primary lesions 1.5–4.0 millimeters in depth is needed even for patients with primary lesions that extend deeper than 4.0 millimeters, as long as the patients show no symptoms suggestive of possible spread of disease. This is because there is no evidence to date that early detection of the spread of melanoma prior to the development of symptoms or physical abnormalities results in a better outcome.

This concept is frequently difficult for patients and their families to understand, since they have so often heard that the key to effective cancer treatment is finding and treating it early. Indeed, we have emphasized exactly that point in our discussions of moles and early melanoma. There is no question that prompt removal of questionable skin lesions to prevent the development of melanoma or to catch it while it is confined to the upper layers of the skin is the most effective protection against the disease. The issue here is quite different, however. Once melanoma has spread from the primary site on the skin, it is very likely that melanoma cells are present in other areas of the body, even though they may not be detectable by any of the modern blood tests or imaging tests currently available. It usually requires at least one billion cells (a tumor 1 centimeter across) before cancer can be detected by these tests. Unfortunately, once even a few melanoma cells are present in other parts of the body, there is usually little medical science can do to prevent recurrence of the disease.

Nevertheless, many patients still want to know from the outset whether or not there is evidence of internal spread of their cancer, since this significantly alters their life expectancy (for better or worse). For this reason, most patients with advanced primary melanomas (greater than 4.0 millimeters) do have more extensive staging studies as part of their initial evaluation. There are differences of opinion among experts as to which tests, if any, are the most useful. For evaluating the lungs, abdomen, and pelvic regions, computerized tomography (CT) scans, which use a combination of X-ray and computer analysis, are currently used most frequently, whereas magnetic resonance imaging (MRI) scans, which use computer-controlled radio waves and magnetic fields, have proven more sensitive for evaluating the brain.

In recent years, doctors have also begun using nuclear medicine studies known as **PET scans** and **gallium scans.** Both of these techniques use a radioisotope that is injected into a vein and, in theory, should be taken up by cancer cells but not by normal cells. The whole body is then scanned with a radiation counter to produce an X-ray-like picture in which areas that have taken up the radioisotope appear as lighted spots. Whether these tests will prove superior to CT or MRI scans for detecting small metastases remains to be proven.

TREATMENT DECISIONS: WHAT RESEARCH STUDIES TELL US

The best initial treatment for patients with advanced melanoma is unclear, and experts often disagree on the best way to manage the disease. Unfortunately, sometimes this means that a confused and frustrated patient is left without reliable professional advice to make a very difficult decision about a very important matter. Because so much remains to be learned about treating patients with melanoma and because there are a number of areas of controversy where patients may have to decide among different treatment options, this is a good place for us to explain medical research studies in some detail. By understanding how these studies are conducted and what you can and cannot learn from them, you will be in a better position to evaluate the advice you receive and make the decision that is right for you.

Oncology (the study and care of patients with cancer) is a unique area of medicine, in that despite years of research, oncologists' ability to treat patients effectively is limited. Cancer remains a most difficult and challenging foe. Great strides have been made in recent decades in the treatment of childhood leukemia, Hodgkin's disease, and testicular cancer, but much more remains to be done. As a result, *clinical trials* (research) form the foundation of cancer management, and new studies are being designed all the time, all over the world, for every type of cancer. Once one trial is completed, a new one is usually designed based on its results—all with the goal of improving the prognosis of patients with cancer.

There are two broad categories of research studies—**prospective** and **retrospective** clinical trials. A prospective trial is carefully planned and designed ahead of time, and patients are recruited to participate in the trial and to be followed closely by the study investigators. A retrospective trial, in contrast, is one done "after the fact." No patients are enrolled in a retrospective trial. Instead, medical records of patients' treatment and follow-up care are reviewed, often many years later.

Prospective Studies

We will begin with prospective trials. The seeds of a clinical trial are sown when a physician or a medical research scientist has an idea that some form of treatment, say a new drug, will be beneficial. The first step is to test the drug in the laboratory using artificially grown cells or animal models. If the results are promising, and the drug appears to be safe, the scientist may propose testing it in humans.

Let's say we want to answer the question of whether our drug can shrink or eliminate melanoma tumors. There are two ways to carry out this prospective trial: an **uncontrolled trial** and a **controlled trial.** In an uncontrolled trial of our hypothetical drug, all of the patients enrolled in the study would be given the drug and then followed to determine the number who have experienced shrinkage of their tumors. These results would then be compared with the outcomes for a *historical control group*—that is, patients with similar tumors who were seen and followed by the same or different doctors at some time in the past and did not receive the drug under study.

At first glance, an uncontrolled trial seems like a reasonable approach. After all, because the drug was found to be beneficial in preliminary laboratory studies, most patients will want to try it. The problem is that the historical patients and the patients receiving the new drug are not truly comparable. The physicians who examined and treated the "historical" patients may be different from those examining and treating the current patients; new and better diagnostic techniques may now be available; surgical techniques may have been improved; methods of follow-up may be different; and the patient mix may have changed. If patients taking the drug appear to do better than their historical counterparts, it may be the result of some or all of these factors rather than the effect of the drug. Uncontrolled trials are often done initially, however, to provide some evidence of benefit to justify doing a larger, more expensive controlled trial.

In a controlled trial, patients are asked to participate knowing that they may or may not get the experimental treatment. It is important to realize that drugs or other therapies showing positive results in the laboratory, including results from tests on experimental animals, do not always prove effective when tested in people. If they did, there would be no point in doing the studies in humans. Study results sometimes show that patients receiving experimental treatments do no better or even do worse than their untreated counterparts. For this reason, it is not true that patients *not* receiving the experimental drug or procedure are necessarily receiving an inferior treatment.

Patients enrolled in the trial are assigned randomly to two or more groups, most often by a computer. (Thus, such trials are often referred to as "randomized trials.") Neither doctor nor patient has any choice over which group the patient will be assigned to, but in almost all cancer trials all patients are informed of what group they are in and what drugs they will be given. One group is the **control** group; the other group(s) is the *experimental group*. Patients in the control group receive the best treatment available at the time the study is designed, but they do not receive the experimental drug or procedure. In some studies, controls are not treated or are given a **placebo** (a pill that looks like the experimental drug but does not contain any medication), but this is unusual in cancer studies. Different dosages of the drug under study may be given to different experimental groups in order to determine side effects and what dosage is most effective.

Various means are used to ensure that the groups are as similar as possible. For example, they should have equal, or close to equal, numbers of males and females, similar patient ages, and similar stages of cancer. Likewise, the follow-up schedule and testing are identical for all members of the study. Although the final results of long-term studies are not known for months or years, preliminary results are analyzed on a regular basis. If members of the experimental groups in a drug test begin to show dangerous side effects, the study will be discontinued. Likewise, if preliminary results of the study show that the drug is clearly effective, it will be offered to the patients in the control group as well.

Many trials of cancer medication are organized by large cooperative oncology groups—for example, the World Health Organization Melanoma Group—that recruit patients from many different participating centers. This is because the number of participants in the trial must be large enough to make the results reliable. At the end of the trial, researchers compare the outcomes of the groups. Rigid statistical analysis of the data ensures that any differences observed by the researchers are due to the drug being studied, and not to chance alone. This is why it is important that the trials be large. If only a few people are being studied, it is difficult to know if the difference in outcome of one or two subjects is due to chance or to the medication being tested.

Differences that are so marked that they cannot be due to chance are called **statistically significant** differences. The medical community accepts only statistically significant findings. Insurance companies are also increasingly limiting coverage to therapies that have been well tested. Although painfully slow at times, well-designed controlled trials are preferable to the delays and false hopes often generated by uncontrolled studies.

Retrospective Studies

Now to retrospective trials. A retrospective study cannot be used to test a new drug, because investigations of *new* treatments cannot, by definition, be done in a retrospective fashion. Retrospective studies are used only to explore the effectiveness of treatments that have been in use for some time. As an example, let's look at the question of whether having the regional lymph nodes that drain the area of your primary melanoma removed at the time you are diagnosed with the disease ("up front" lymph node **dissection**) is more effective than removing the lymph nodes only if they become enlarged over time (the "watch and wait" approach). This is a very real question, which we will discuss further below.

The quickest and easiest (but not the most definitive) way to approach this question is to use "old" patients—that is, patients who have already had a lymph node dissection done some years ago. Patients who had their lymph node dissection done up front, for whatever reason, are compared with patients from a similar time period who, also for whatever reason, had their lymph nodes removed only if they became enlarged over time. Patients from each group are selected, and their records are reviewed by the investigators to determine which group did better. Some or all of the patients in the study may never have been cared for by the doctors conducting the study. This is a retrospective study.

The retrospective approach can be useful. It is often from the examination of historical records that questions are raised for testing in prospective controlled studies. Relying on retrospective studies alone, however, is fraught with problems. As with uncontrolled prospective trials, the equality of the historical "control" group and the historical "experimental" group cannot be assured. You can imagine, for example, that some of the patients who did not undergo lymph node dissection at the time of diagnosis were elderly or were suffering from other illnesses, and that is why the watch and wait approach was adopted by the patient or the physician. Indeed, factors such as this will without a doubt influence outcome and may lead to conclusions that are later disproved by a randomized controlled study.

Another concern with retrospective studies is that it is easy for an investigator to introduce his or her own bias unintentionally when selecting patients for inclusion in the study. Say you are a surgeon and your preconceived notion, based on your own experience, is that patients who have a lymph node dissection up front do better than those who adopt the watch and wait approach. It is easy—without conscious intent—to create selection criteria that will sway the results in favor of your bias.

What's the bottom line on clinical trials? The bottom line is that, although other research trials can provide useful information, only carefully designed, prospective, randomized, controlled trials with large numbers of patients can be trusted to yield reliable results. It is also important to recognize that premature reports of fantastic new cancer treatments or even cures are frequently released to the media well before any true test results are in. Such reports may, for example, be based on the results of preliminary laboratory tests. Other seemingly exciting news may turn out to have been obtained from poorly designed studies with very small numbers of patients. A good rule of thumb is to be skeptical of any new treatments you read or hear about until you can discuss the claims with a melanoma specialist.

EVALUATION AND TREATMENT OF REGIONAL LYMPH NODES AT THE TIME OF DIAGNOSIS

Now that we have discussed research studies, we can look at how they have been applied to the question of how best to treat primary melanomas. Because the goal of this treatment is to prevent recurrence of the disease, one area that physicians have focused on is the lymph nodes. In the past it was believed that melanoma cells spread in a very systematic fashion, first from the site of origin to the lymph nodes that drained the area of the original lesion and then—and only then—to the internal organs. This led to the widely held belief that if the draining lymph nodes were removed, the cancer could not spread. Based on this theory, all patients with newly diagnosed melanoma underwent an **elective regional lymph node dissection.** ("Elective" means the operation was done, not out of medical necessity, but rather, to try to improve the outcome.)

In this procedure, all of the lymph nodes in the region most likely to drain the site of the primary tumor were surgically removed, whether or not they were thought to contain metastatic melanoma cells at the time of surgery. Physicians later realized, however, that removal of the lymph nodes in this way did not always prevent the subsequent appearance of melanoma in other organs, and that some patients developed metastases in their internal organs without ever having melanoma in their lymph nodes. This realization, of course, called into question the use of elective regional lymph node dissection.

These observations led to several large retrospective research studies in which patients who had had regional lymph node dissections at the time of diagnosis (up front) were compared with those who had had their lymph nodes removed only when and if they became enlarged, suggesting they contained metastatic melanoma cells (the wait and see approach). Many of these studies suggested that patients undergoing elective regional lymph node dissection when they were first diagnosed with melanoma may do a bit better than patients choosing the watch and wait approach, but they showed no overwhelming advantage. Based on these results, two large prospective randomized controlled trials involving several different medical centers were designed to answer the question definitively.

In contrast to the earlier retrospective studies, both of the prospective trials demonstrated that patients who underwent lymph node dissection as soon as their melanoma was diagnosed did not live longer than patients who underwent lymph node dissection only when their lymph nodes became enlarged. In other words, many patients in the first group underwent a major operation for no apparent benefit. There was a suggestion, however, from one of these large prospective studies that elective lymph node dissection did benefit patients under age 60 who had primary lesions 1–4 millimeters thick. These patients had a higher likelihood of having melanoma cells in their lymph nodes, even if the nodes did not appear to be enlarged. The problem was that there were not enough patients in this category to say for sure.

Similar cooperative studies are now under way to answer this question once and for all. These studies are enrolling only patients with deep primaries (1.5 millimeters or greater) and lymph nodes that are not enlarged at diagnosis. The results of one of these studies from the World Health Organization Melanoma Program were released in March 1998. This study showed that for all patients taken together, elective lymph node dissection did not improve outcome.

The goal has now become the identification of patients who have microscopic deposits of melanoma (**micrometastases**) in their lymph nodes before they undergo a complete lymph node dissection. This is being done with the techniques of lymphoscintigraphy and sentinel node biopsy. (These techniques are discussed in the next section of this chapter.) This approach allows the surgeon to select only those patients with melanoma in the lymph nodes for further lymph node dissection, sparing those whose nodes are free of melanoma. New methods for detecting these micrometastases are being developed. When completed, these studies should provide clear guidance for doctors and patients about the potential benefits of this major operation. For the moment, we would advise regional lymph node dissection for patients with primary melanomas deeper than 1 millimeter and clinically negative (not enlarged) lymph nodes only if done with lymphoscintigraphy and sentinel node biopsy.

Tammy's Story

When Tammy's orthopedist mentioned that a mole on her neck looked too dark for her skin tone, the 31-year-old mother of two small children did not pay much attention. She didn't have time, she said, for "something that didn't hurt, bleed, or cry."

When her dermatologist removed the mole, sent it to a pathologist, and referred her to an oncologist, however, he got her attention. The report said "Clark's level IV melanoma." The oncologist explained that because of the melanoma's proximity to the lymph nodes in the neck, Tammy would need radical surgery involving a 7-inch incision from the ear lobe to the middle of the neck, with removal of the lymph nodes and a resultant large scar and indentation. Tammy questioned him extensively on the procedure, and they scheduled surgery for four days later. When she left his office, she felt numb, but she also had a copy of the pathologist's report.

During the next two days, Tammy solicited second opinions by faxing her report to oncologists across the United States. Most agreed with her doctor that the surgery was the proper next step to prevent recurrence. Finally, she faxed the report to a research physician recommended by a friend. He dissented, and he substantiated his stance with years of research documenting the ineffectiveness of the surgery. Tammy's doctor was irritated, but he agreed to consult a doctor from a major melanoma research center. Tammy recounts the result: "The next morning, I received a call that was one of the most enlightened moments I've had. My surgeon had spoken with the research hospital, and after 'much review,' he no longer recommended the surgery. He had reconsidered based on 'new evidence and data' they had shared with him. I was so relieved, but I realized that without significant efforts on my part (and the help of many), I would have undergone an extensive surgical procedure that was no longer recommended."

Lymphoscintigraphy and Sentinel Node Biopsy

In the past, surgeons performing elective regional lymph node dissections on patients with a primary melanoma on the face, back, abdomen, or chest faced a difficult challenge. Unless the patient had enlarged lymph nodes suggestive of lymph node metastases, it was not easy to know which lymph nodes to remove because several lymph node chains may drain any of these sites. For example, as mentioned earlier, a primary melanoma on the middle of the back might drain to lymph nodes in either of the armpits or groin regions or to either side of the neck or collarbone regions. For years, surgeons relied on drawings of the human lymphatic system made in the last century to guide them as to which lymph nodes to remove (see Figure 7.1).

A new technique known as **lymphoscintigraphy** is now available, however, to help remove the guesswork about which lymph nodes are responsible for draining the region of any given primary. In recent years, the popularity of this technique has soared, and it is quickly becoming the standard of care in evaluating lymph nodes in patients with deep primary lesions (deeper than 1 millimeter) and non-enlarged lymph nodes.

In lymphoscintigraphy, the doctor injects a small amount of a radioactive tracer into the skin around the site of the primary lesion. The tracer is taken up by the body's lymphatic channels, which in turn empty into lymph node basins. Using nuclear medicine scans, the doctor is able to detect the presence of the radioactive tracer in the draining lymph nodes. This novel technique has led to many surprises and demonstrated that the previously relied upon lymphatic maps are often completely inaccurate. For example, while the maps would predict that a melanoma on the left lower back would drain to the left groin, lymphoscintigraphy might reveal that the actual drainage was to the right groin or sometimes to even less predictable sites, such as the neck.

After lymphoscintigraphy has defined the lymph node area draining the primary melanoma, new techniques known as **intraoperative lymphatic mapping** and **sentinel node biopsy** are used to determine if melanoma cells are present. The **sentinel lymph node** is the first lymph node seen to take up the radioactive tracer in the lymphoscintigraphy procedure. In the new approach to making decisions about surgery, lymphoscintigraphy is followed by a minor surgical procedure known as intraoperative lymphatic mapping. This is done in the operating room under general anesthesia. First, a special blue dye is injected into the site of the primary melanoma. Then the lymph node basin shown by lymphoscintigraphy to contain the sentinel lymph node is prepared for surgery, and a one-half-inch to one-inch cut is made in that area so that the blue-stained sentinel lymph node can be found. The sentinel lymph node is then removed and immediately examined microscopically by a pathologist. If the sentinel node is found to contain melanoma cells, then a formal lymph node dissection is performed. If the sentinel node shows no evidence of melanoma, then the patient is spared the lymph node dissection procedure.

For now, most specialists recommend that patients with primary melanomas invading 1 millimeter or more, but without enlarged lymph nodes at the time of diagnosis, undergo lymphoscintigraphy followed by intraoperative lymphatic mapping and sentinel node biopsy. Patients found to have melanoma in the sentinel lymph node should then undergo formal lymph node dissection, while those with a negative sentinel node biopsy need not. Because this technology is so new, large prospective trials evaluating its benefit have not yet been completed. What has been shown is that the micrometastases detected in this way carry with them a worse prognosis than would be the case if no melanoma cells had been found. This has meant that these patients can be targeted for more careful follow-up and for new adjuvant therapies now being tested (see Chapter 9).

Other Cases

We have discussed extensively the management of lymph nodes in patients with primary melanomas that are at least 1 millimeter in depth without enlarged lymph nodes at diagnosis. What about patients with thinner primaries as well as patients with enlarged lymph nodes at diagnosis? Even the strongest advocates for elective lymph node dissection agree that patients with primary melanomas less than 1.0 millimeters deep do not benefit from the procedure, because their likelihood of cure without any further treatment is so high. Likewise, even the strongest critics of up-front lymph node dissection agree that patients with enlarged lymph nodes shown to contain melanoma at the time of diagnosis do benefit from early lymph node dissection.

"Enlarged" means the lymph nodes can be felt by the patient or physician. Remember, lymph nodes can be enlarged for reasons other than melanoma. They often become enlarged when we are fighting off an infection. In order to determine whether enlarged lymph nodes contain melanoma, the physician will perform a **fine needle aspiration** (FNA). (This procedure can only be done on enlarged lymph nodes.) The FNA is an office procedure done with a needle and syringe, much like taking a blood sample. Anesthesia is not usually required, though some physicians use a small injection of a novocaine-like drug. The needle is inserted into the lymph node several times while the plunger on the syringe is pulled back, sucking cells into it. The cells in the syringe are then pushed out onto a glass slide, dyed with special stains, and studied by a pathologist. A diagnosis can usually be made within 30 minutes of the procedure, and the results are accurate. If melanoma is found, the next step is a regional lymph node dissection.

PROGNOSIS AND FOLLOW-UP

Prognosis means the expected outlook for a patient with a disease. For patients who have had a lesion removed that has been diagnosed as melanoma, prognosis means the likelihood that the tumor will come back and spread to the internal organs, and if so when. Statistics for melanoma, like all cancers, have been generated on the basis of careful long-term follow-up of thousands of patients with all stages of the disease. The people compiling these statistics collect detailed information about patients at the time their melanoma was diagnosed. They then monitor the same patients closely over many years, keeping track of when and if recurrences or death occurred. As you would expect, the higher the stage of the melanoma, the more likely it is to recur later.

With all stages, there are persons who survive regardless of the odds and statistics. It is impossible to predict the outcome for any given individual; one can only provide the odds. The odds are usually given in 5- or 10-year survival graphs. These show the percentage of people still alive after 5 or 10 years on one axis and the characteristic being studied (original diagnosis, age at diagnosis, specific treatment, etc.) on the other. A 10-year survival graph for melanoma patients is shown in Figure 8.1. It is based on the Clark's level and Breslow depth of the primary lesion at the time of diagnosis.

Although the stage at diagnosis is by far the most powerful factor influencing the prognosis in melanoma patients (the lower the stage, the better the outlook), predicted outcome can be further refined by taking into account a number of other **prognostic factors.** For example, women who have not yet gone through menopause tend to have a lower chance for recurrence than women who have gone through menopause and a lower chance than men. The reasons behind this are not clear. Lack of ulceration or bleeding of the primary lesion, melanoma on the front of the arms or the legs, and a low growth rate (called the mitotic index) as determined by the pathologist are all associated with a better prognosis. Melanoma located in what has been called the **BANS** region (the **b**ack and the back of the **a**rms, **n**eck, and **s**houlders) has been associated with a worse prognosis, probably because these places are all hard to see, so diagnosis tends to occur late.

Follow-up refers to the frequency and type of medical examinations and tests following the diagnosis (or suspicion) of a disease. After a diagnosis of melanoma, two of the most commonly asked questions are, "How often will I have to have a checkup?" and "What will be done to determine if the melanoma has come back?" There are no rules engraved in stone, but a guideline is that *all patients should have follow-up.* The type and frequency required depends mainly on the stage at diagnosis.

There are two reasons you need to have periodic evaluations if you have had melanoma. The first is that people who have had one melanoma are at risk of developing another; their risk of non-melanoma skin cancer is also increased. This is because the factors that caused the first melanoma (usually a lot of sun exposure and genetic predisposition) can never be erased, and people who have had a melanoma at one site usually have damage to melanocytes in other

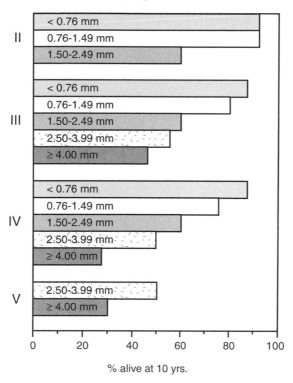

FIGURE 8.1. Ten-year survival. Estimated percentage of patients surviving for ten years with primary melanomas of various Clark's levels and Breslow's depths of invasion. Note that, for all Clark's levels, the depth in millimeters may vary based upon the site of the melanoma, on the body, age, and sex of the patient, and on other factors. In general the deeper the melanoma, the higher the death rate. Survival for level one patients is one hundred percent (assuming the biopsy is read correctly). Level II lesions are rarely greater than 2.5 millimeters and level V lesions are rarely less than 2.5 millimeters, so there are not accurate statistics available for these cases.

areas as well. The risk for a second melanoma is not high—1 to 5%—but it should not be ignored, especially since melanoma is almost always completely curable when detected early. People with an inherited predisposition to melanoma have a much higher risk of developing a second primary, and many such people will develop many melanomas unless they are extremely vigilant.

Once you have been diagnosed with melanoma, you should have your doctor perform a very thorough examination of every nook and cranny of your skin (including between the toes, on the scalp, and in the genital areas) looking for other suspicious moles that should also be removed. Find a physician with experience in melanoma who will examine all of your skin completely and thoroughly, not only at the time of diagnosis, but at every follow-up visit.

The second reason for follow-up examinations is to determine if there is any evidence that the melanoma has spread to the lymph nodes or internal organs. Although early detection of recurrence has not been correlated statistically with a better prognosis, it is our view that all patients with a diagnosis of invasive melanoma (Clark's levels II to V) deserve periodic evaluation by a doctor, since earlier diagnosis and treatment of internal organ involvement may occasionally lead to cure and can prevent pain and suffering. Everyone who has treated large numbers of patients with melanoma can remember patients who had a single lung or brain metastasis and were cured by surgical removal of the tumor.

The studies used to follow patients with melanoma are the doctor's physical examination, blood tests, X rays, and scans. All patients should have a careful physical examination at each visit, with particular attention to the site of the original melanoma and the skin around that site, the lymph nodes, the lungs, and the liver. Specific complaints, such as unexplained pain, may direct the physician to further examination of a particular area. Blood tests are used to determine the function of internal organs such as the liver. X rays of the chest are used to check the lungs, and other scans are used to evaluate the other internal organs and the brain.

Doctors disagree about when and how often each of these should be done. For patients with stage I melanoma, a physical examination every 6–12 months for 5 years is generally all that is required, since the likelihood of cure is so high. Patients who have stage II melanoma require more careful follow-up dictated by their individual cases. For example, was it a thinner or deeper stage II lesion? Was it on the extremities or in the BANS region? Is the patient a man or a young woman? And so on. For this group of patients as a whole, we would advise (at a minimum) that for 5 years the patient have a physical examination every 6–12 months, a complete blood count including liver function tests yearly, and an annual chest X ray. If any of these tests uncover abnormalities or if the patient has unexplained symptoms, further testing with scans or biopsies may be needed.

Stage III patients require more diligent follow-up, since 75% will eventually develop a recurrence. We advise physical examinations every 3–4 months for the first 2 years, every 6 months for the next 3 years, and yearly thereafter. This is because the likelihood of recurrence for these patients gradually tapers off with time, but it never becomes zero. During the 5 years after their initial diagnosis, these patients should have blood tests every 6 months and a chest X ray, whole body CT or PET scan, and brain MRI scan every year. After 5 years, it is reasonable to limit the testing to annual blood tests and chest X rays, provided the patient has no symptoms and there are no abnormal findings on the physical examination.

Patients with stage IV melanoma already have metastases. Their follow-up will depend on the extent and site of their tumors, symptoms or abnormalities revealed by physical examinations or blood tests, and the type of treatment they are receiving.

Again, let us remind you that these are general guidelines only. As the worldwide effort to limit health care costs grows, insurance plans are likely to be increasingly reluctant to cover extensive testing in patients who feel completely well. If you cannot have all of the tests recommended above, your prognosis will probably not be affected. If you do develop any symptoms, however, it is important that you get sufficient testing to explain them.

As you can see, the treatment goal for all primary melanomas that have not invaded the internal organs is to remove all detectable melanoma cells. In the next chapter, we will discuss a wide variety of therapies that are being developed to address the question of whether there is anything that can be done to help prevent recurrence of melanoma after wide local excision and lymph node surgery. These are called **adjuvant therapies.**

9

. . .

Adjuvant Therapy

We know from research studies that many people who are diagnosed with either stage II or stage III melanoma are probably harboring microscopic cancer cells (micrometastases) that may later show up as detectable metastases. (Their rate of recurrence is shown in Figure 8.1.) In these studies, patients had wide local excision of their primary lesions either alone or in combination with lymph node dissection, and at the end of the initial treatment and staging, they had no detectable evidence of melanoma in the rest of their bodies. Some of these people, however, later had a recurrence of their melanoma. We have already seen in preceding chapters that the presence of undetectable micrometastases is a common and difficult problem in both melanoma and other cancers. In hopes of getting rid of these micrometastases before they have a chance to grow and cause problems, cancer specialists often give these patients adjuvant therapy (literally, "helping" or "enhancing" therapy). Researchers have studied many different forms of adjuvant therapy for melanoma patients and are currently testing others. Among the approaches being explored are immunotherapy, radiation therapy, chemotherapy, vitamins, and psychotherapy, either alone or in various combinations. We will discuss each of these in some detail.

IMMUNOTHERAPY

The term **immunotherapy** encompasses many different forms of treatment, all of which have the goal of harnessing the body's immune system to attack disease—in this case, residual melanoma cells. Researchers are especially hopeful that immunotherapy may be an

Melanoma research is littered with the remains of hundreds of uncontrolled trials of adjuvant therapies. Both patients and doctors are so eager to find a therapy that will *A word of caution about unproven therapies* prevent recurrence that they sometimes overreact to rumors or premature suggestions that an effective therapy has been found. Remember that no therapy is proven to be beneficial until it has been evaluated using rigorous scientific testing methods with proper control groups. This means that any new treatment must be tested in a controlled fashion—either compared to no treatment or compared to the best known treatment that has been proven to be beneficial.

Even when studies have been concluded, their results may be less clearcut than we might hope. For example, a therapy might prove to be beneficial to 20–30% of a given group of patients—not a total success, but better than none. Of course, studies take time, and doctors sometimes prescribe "promising" therapies so long as their side effects do not seem serious.

Deciding what adjuvant therapy is right for you will involve balancing its possible side effects against its likelihood of success. Such decisions should always be made in collaboration with your physician. Get a second or even third opinion if you feel uncertain of the right course. Never be shy about asking questions, and never rush into an unproven therapy without consultation. It may prove to have dangers you are unaware of, or it simply may not be the most effective therapy available.

effective treatment for melanoma because occasionally patients' melanoma metastases get smaller or disappear spontaneously, without medical treatment. The change is presumably brought about by the patient's own immune system. These cases are few and far between, but they have sparked the imagination of research scientists for generations and have led to hundreds of studies over the past 50 years.

Immunotherapy studies are based on the premise that, for unknown reasons, the immune systems of melanoma patients are unable to recognize melanoma cells as abnormal or foreign. A healthy immune system recognizes the cells that are part of our bodies and leaves them alone. When viruses, parasites, bacteria, or other organisms enter our bodies, however, a healthy immune system recognizes them as foreign and mounts an elaborate immune response to destroy them. Researchers have reasoned that if the immune systems of melanoma patients could be made to recognize the melanoma cells as foreign invaders, the melanoma could be eliminated by natural means. Unfortunately, this has proved to be much easier said than done.

Nonspecific Immunotherapy

The first attempts at immunotherapy used nonspecific stimulants to boost the immune system generally, rather than agents that

A few words about the immune response

The immune response is an extremely complicated process in which many of our body's cells and proteins play important parts. Scientists are still unraveling its intricacies. We hope this overview will help you better understand the research studies and treatment options you may hear about.

All cells carry proteins known as **antigens** on their surfaces. These proteins have a variety of functions; one of them is recognition. All the antigens on the cells that are native to our bodies have specific components that identify them as belonging to us (as being "self"). The antigens on the surfaces of foreign microorganisms that invade our bodies have different configurations ("nonself").

There are many different kinds of cells in our immune system. All carry receptor proteins on their surfaces that distinguish between "self" and "nonself." Some of these immune cells carry receptor proteins called **antibodies** whose job is to recognize only one specific foreign antigen, such as an antigen on a particular flu virus. These immune cells can also release antibodies into the bloodstream. When an antibody comes in contact with its specific antigen, the antibody, whether bound to a cell or freely circulating, binds to the specific antigen, beginning a cascade of events whose purpose is to destroy all the microorganisms in our bodies that carry that antigen. One of the important things that happens during a normal *immune response* is that the binding of antibody to antigen stimulates the proliferation of other immune cells, which move in to kill the foreign invader. This means that your immune system becomes specialized in finding and destroying that particular organism.

would focus it specifically on melanoma cells. These nonspecific immunotherapies included multiple injections of the tuberculosis vaccine BCG, a bacterial agent called *C. parvum,* a drug called levamisole that is normally used to treat intestinal worms, and a host of other agents. On the basis of small, uncontrolled trials, these agents were touted enthusiastically as means of reducing the risk of a recurrence of melanoma. This enthusiasm, however, quickly gave way to skepticism after carefully controlled trials in which these agents were compared with placebos or no treatment in comparable patient groups showed no benefit. Nonspecific immunotherapy is still practiced, but only by a few diehards. Agents that stimulate the overall immune system are sometimes used in conjunction with a more directed approach, however.

Tumor-Specific Immunotherapy

With the realization that nonspecific immunotherapy was unlikely to be as effective as they had hoped, investigators turned to making *melanoma-specific* **vaccines.** Vaccines for infectious diseases like measles are preparations, usually containing dead or at least noninfectious organisms, which are given to people to produce or increase an immune response to that organism. A large number of melanoma-specific vaccines have been tested, or are currently being tested, in humans. The basic idea is to identify an **antigen** that is made only by melanoma cells, not by any of the normal cells of the body, and to make a vaccine against it.

Melanoma cells usually do not make truly foreign proteins, since they arise from the body's own cells, but they often make proteins or antigens that are unique to them and are not present on normal melanocytes or other body cells. Antigens that are unique to cancer cells are called *tumor-specific antigens.* The objective of tumor-specific immunotherapy is to make a vaccine against a tumor-specific antigen that will rally the immune system against the tumor cells. Again, this has proved to be much easier said than done.

Initially scientists used crude extracts of killed melanoma cells to make the vaccines. More recently, improved technology has allowed researchers to identify and purify melanoma-specific antigens in the laboratory to provide more specific vaccines. These are called *peptide vaccines.* They are usually given in multiple injections under the skin, and since the tumor-specific antigens are not truly foreign, they are often given together with other agents like smallpox vaccines to make them more "attractive" to the immune system.

Again, despite great enthusiasm, hope, and hype, none of these vaccines has as yet been shown to have a statistically significant long-term benefit in controlled trials. For one thing, the immune system is not so easily fooled: Added agents (such as smallpox vaccine) have not fully overcome the immune system's reluctance to attack cells whose antigens are not truly foreign. Also, not all melanoma cells in a given patient make the same antigens, so even if a patient's immune system does attack and kill some melanoma cells, many cells may be missed.

For many years researchers believed that once a cancer (any cancer) developed, all of the cells derived from the original cancer cell would be exactly the same, and that all of the cells arising from them would, in turn, be identical (see the description of clones in Chapter 3). We now know that this is far from the case. Rather, as cancer cells grow and divide, they continually mutate or change. In a single patient with metastatic melanoma, there may be hundreds or even thousands of different clones of cells. They all began from an initial cell, but over time, they change, just as the human population is now very different from our early ancestors. Although these different cell clones are all still recognizable as melanoma, they are as different as people from different cultures because of mutations that arise with cell proliferation. It remains to be seen whether any of the many current trials of tumor-specific immunotherapy will live up to their proclaimed potential. So far, tumor-specific vaccines are available only as part of clinical trials.

Cytokines

Cytokines are chemical signals. They are proteins made in one cell that regulate the activity of other cells. They can trigger proliferation in immune cells and attract these additional cells to the site where they are needed. When you get an infection on your skin, for example, cytokines are made and released from the area, circulating in the blood and lymph systems and announcing to the body that help is needed. Cytokines aid attacking immune cells by signaling them to proliferate rapidly, telling them where to go, enlarging the blood vessels to expedite their travel to the site of trouble, and assisting in the cleanup. A large number of different cytokines have been discovered during the past 20 years. Among those you might have heard or read about are interferons, interleukins, colony-stimulating factors, tumor necrosis factor, and endothelins. More are being discovered every day. Many cytokines have been purified and can now be produced in large enough quantities for treatment of human diseases. The two that have been most widely studied for the treatment of melanoma are **alpha interferon** and **interleukin 2.**

ALPHA INTERFERON

There are three major interferons—alpha, beta, and gamma. They are called interferons because they were originally discovered as proteins that interfered with viral infection of cells grown in the laboratory. All of these forms of interferon are produced naturally by immune cells in the body when a viral infection has occurred, presumably to help fight off the infection. In fact, the body's own production of interferon in response to the flu virus, not the virus itself, is what causes you to feel so ill when you get the flu.

All three forms of interferon have been tested for activity against human melanoma, but only the alpha form has consistently demonstrated some benefit in the treatment of melanoma patients and has been approved for use as both adjuvant therapy and for the treatment of advanced disease. Despite almost 20 years of study, it is still not entirely clear exactly how alpha interferon works in melanoma.

Injections of alpha interferon are known to alter the surface of melanoma cells, making them easier for the immune system to recognize. They also increase the number of immune system cells and make them more active. While these actions are not in any way specific for melanoma—again, it is just a general revving up of the immune system—they do seem to work in some cases.

The subjects of the initial alpha interferon studies were people with melanoma that had already spread. The researchers tested different dosages and routes of administration (intravenous and under-the-skin injections). The results were less spectacular than the researchers had hoped. Nonetheless, about 20% of the people receiving alpha interferon had regression of their melanoma, and a few have still not had a recurrence more than 10 years later.

The people who responded to the interferon were most often those who had only limited spread of the disease at the time they were treated—those with subcutaneous nodules only or those whose melanoma was restricted to the lymph nodes or the lungs. People whose melanoma had spread to many organs usually did not respond. This probably reflects what we learned earlier: the more widespread the melanoma is, the more likely it is to have developed "multiple faces" as the result of mutations over time. Some of the melanoma clones may be killed with the aid of interferon, but some may not. Unfortunately, it only takes a single clone of melanoma cells to cause problems. Recognition of this problem led to the idea that earlier treatment with interferon in patients who were at high risk for recurrence might have the greatest benefit.

About 10 years ago, researchers began trials of alpha interferon as an adjuvant therapy. Again, the study designs included a large number of different doses and schedules of administration. In the largest controlled trial to date, by the U.S. Eastern Cooperative Oncology Group (ECOG), more than 600 patients with advanced stage II (greater than 4 millimeters) and stage III melanoma (see Chapter 8) were randomly assigned to a control group and an experimental group. Both groups had their primary and regional lymph nodes removed—standard treatment at the time. Controls received no further treatment (also standard). Subjects in the treatment group received large intravenous doses of alpha interferon (20 million units [MU] per meter-squared) for one month, followed by doses of 10 MUs per meter-squared, which they administered to themselves under the skin three times a week for 48 weeks.

In the ECOG study, patients with stage III and advanced stage II (greater than 4 millimeters) melanoma whose primary melanoma and lymph nodes had been removed surgically were treated with alpha interferon to try to prevent recurrence (adjuvant therapy) and compared with an untreated control group. In an early evaluation of this study, in 1996, the treated group showed a slight but statistically significant reduction in recurrence and death from melanoma in com-

Meter-squared is a commonly used means of determining the dose of a drug, particularly in oncology. Using the patient's height and weight, a calculation is made of the body's entire surface area in meters squared, just as a carpenter would determine the surface area of a room. The average-sized adult has a surface area of just under 2 square meters. Using meter-squared measurements is more accurate than using weight alone to calculate drug dosage and ensures that all patients get approximately the same dose proportionate to their size.

Patients come in so many sizes, how can researchers be sure that study patients are all receiving the same dose of medicine?

parison with the nontreated group. The results were not dramatic, however: After 4 years, 70% of the patients treated in the standard fashion had died, compared to 60% of the patients treated with alpha interferon. Analysis of the results showed that patients who had enlarged lymph nodes containing melanoma (stage III disease) before treatment benefited from the treatment, while patients with deep melanomas confined to the skin (the patients with advanced stage II disease) showed no benefit. In 1999, however, a longer-term analysis of this study found that there was no difference in survival between the treated and untreated control groups.

In addition, this high-dosage treatment resulted in a huge number of side effects, and a few deaths were attributed directly to the treatment itself. If you remember that flu symptoms are caused by the body's natural production of interferon, you won't be surprised that the most common side effects included severe fatigue, fever, and a flu-like syndrome. Other common side effects were weight loss and hair loss, anemia, low white blood cell counts, and abnormal liver blood tests. Most of these side effects improved during the course of treatment or resolved when the treatment ended. This was the first carefully controlled adjuvant trial of interferon in a large number of patients and at first seemed to be encouraging.

Unfortunately, long-term study failed to confirm the initial findings. Currently it can be said that there is no evidence to indicate that there is any statistically significant survival benefit to using high-dose alpha interferon as adjuvant therapy in melanoma. At present, its use can be recommended only as part of a clinical research trial. New studies, in which other immunotherapy and chemotherapy agents are added to interferon, are now under way. The results of these studies will not be known for several years.

At the same time that high-dose interferon studies were going on, other investigators from a number of centers around the world were studying lower and less toxic doses of adjuvant interferon given as shots under the skin for stage II and III melanoma patients. These studies are too numerous to mention in detail, but their results have given a similar very mixed picture. The doses used have varied from 3 MUs three times a week for 12 weeks to 3 MUs three times a week for 2 years. Although these doses have indeed been well tolerated with few side effects compared to the doses used in the ECOG study, it is not yet certain whether they will provide any benefit. Some studies have reported a slight benefit, others no benefit at all. Still others have reported that the benefit only lasts during the time of interferon administration, suggesting that patients may have to take it continuously throughout their lives.

In short, all that can be said at this point is that the jury is still out and that the benefit from adjuvant interferon is, at best, small. What these studies point out more than anything else is the need for more innovative and effective adjuvant therapies. We hope some of the therapies now being tested will provide more reliable benefit. (For more information about alpha interferon, see Chapter 10.)

INTERLEUKIN 2

We will say more about interleukin 2 (IL-2) in Chapter 10 when we discuss the treatment of advanced melanoma. Like interferon, IL-2 is a cytokine normally made in the body as part of the immune system's armamentarium (weapons system). IL-2 administration increases the number and fighting power of cells in the immune system known as *T cells* and *natural killer cells*. Like interferon, IL-2 was first tested in patients with advanced melanoma. In these studies, a few patients (less than 20%) responded to the treatment. This led to trials of IL-2 as adjuvant therapy, both alone and in combination with interferon. These studies are not complete, and we do not yet know how effective IL-2 will be as an adjuvant therapy.

RADIATION THERAPY

For many years, it was common practice after removing cancerous lymph nodes to treat the areas with adjuvant radiation therapy to kill any remaining melanoma cells in the area and to prevent spread. This is still done in some treatment centers, although less frequently with the advent of other adjuvant treatments. The current belief is that radiation therapy is most beneficial when there are many lymph nodes involved or they are quite large. Radiation treatment may well reduce the likelihood of local recurrence in the lymph node area, but it is probably of limited or no benefit in reducing the likelihood of melanoma's subsequent spread to the internal organs. And radiation treatment can in itself be troublesome, causing pain and swelling. We will say more about radiation therapy in the following chapter.

CHEMOTHERAPY

There is growing interest in adjuvant chemotherapy for melanoma, and a number of large studies in this area are under way. The delay in using this form of treatment as an adjuvant therapy is due to two factors. First was the difficulty of finding a promising drug to test. Only drugs that showed significant benefit in the treatment of advanced melanoma seemed worth testing, and until recently only a few such drugs had been found. Second were the results of two large and carefully controlled trials of the chemotherapy drug DTIC reported in the 1970s. DTIC has in the past proved beneficial in treating advanced melanoma, but one trial of the drug as an *adjuvant* treatment found that the treated group had a higher recurrence and death rate than the nontreated group.

In recent years, however, there has been slow but significant progress in the treatment of advanced melanoma with new drugs or combinations of drugs with cytokines, and better means of managing the side effects and complications resulting from their administration. Current studies are taking these same agents and combinations into clinical trials as adjuvant therapy for melanoma patients at high risk for recurrence. Early results should be available within the next few years, but until these are known, this form of adjuvant therapy should be considered experimental.

VITAMINS AND DIET

One of the questions most commonly asked by people diagnosed with melanoma is, "What can I eat and what vitamins should I take to prevent the melanoma from coming back?" There has been a great interest in the use of vitamins, especially the so-called antioxidants (vitamins A, E, and C, and beta carotene), to prevent the development or recurrence of all kinds of human cancers. Probably no other area is as filled with myths and pseudoscience. There are books by self-proclaimed experts, Internet sites, personal testimonies, superslick sales pitches, and gimmicks, all backed by a lot of bad and sometimes self-serving science.

If you have been diagnosed with melanoma, you will no doubt be deluged with advice from well-meaning friends and family about what to eat and what vitamins to take. The truth is that no dietary supplement or vitamin has ever been shown to prevent the development or recurrence of melanoma. Despite this fact, almost everyone takes them in some form or another, including the most learned scientists and doctors who have been diagnosed with melanoma. Their rationale is that they will not hurt and could help.

What every good study in this complicated area has shown is that a diet high in fresh fruits and vegetables can reduce the risk for the development of some kinds of cancer. As far as we are aware, however, there have been no studies of the effect of diet on the risk of developing melanoma. There have been a few controlled trials of vitamin A compounds as adjuvant therapy, but they have not shown any benefit.

For the moment, the best that can be said is that a diet rich in fresh fruits and vegetables is likely to be healthful in many ways, but we do not know that it will be beneficial in preventing recurrence of melanoma. In general, it is clear that one cannot substitute a few vitamin pills for a good diet—that is, actually eating fruits and vegetables regularly. Natural foods contain hundreds, perhaps thousands, of compounds (including but not limited to vitamins) that appear to be important to the body.

Finally, a word of caution. High doses of some vitamins, particularly vitamin A, can have serious health consequences, including increased cholesterol and abnormalities in liver function. If you choose to take vitamins or food supplements as part of your adjuvant program, talk with your doctor about it so he or she can both guide you as far as how much to take and take your vitamin intake into account when evaluating the results of physical examinations and blood tests.

Changes in Lifestyle

Another question commonly asked by patients diagnosed with melanoma is, "Doctor, will reducing the stress in my life help prevent my melanoma from coming back?" Again, although a host of books, magazine articles, and TV shows have featured information about how stress reduction can strengthen your immune system to fight off cancer and other diseases, scientific evidence to support this contention is scanty. There is no proof that stress causes melanoma, although almost every patient feels stressed at the time of the diagnosis and can recall significant stress in the months or years before.

There are also claims that certain personality types are more prone to cancer and its recurrence. Even if this is true—and we are far from certain that it is—it is unlikely that long-established patterns of behavior can be changed to influence the outcome of a disease like melanoma. Nevertheless, there is one intriguing study from a major U.S. medical center in which a small group of patients with newly diagnosed melanoma were either randomly assigned to a support group where they received counseling about behavior modification or were left to their own devices. During the 5-year study period, those in the support group had lower recurrence and death rates than those in the control group. The differences were small, however, and the findings need to be confirmed in a larger trial.

Although the effectiveness of stress reduction, a healthy diet, and daily exercise as adjuvant therapies is uncertain, these lifestyle habits are important for your general health and well-being. We recommend these measures to everyone, and if they help even one person avoid or delay the recurrence of melanoma, we will be delighted. Should your melanoma recur, however, you should not blame yourself. It is not likely to be because you did not eat the right foods, exercise enough, or reduce the stress in your life.

Sadly, we have a long way to go in developing adjuvant therapies that prevent the recurrence of most melanomas. In the next chapter we will look at what we can and cannot do for patients with advanced disease.

10

Treating Advanced Melanoma

I f your melanoma was diagnosed as Clark's level I and all the margins were clear when the site was re-excised, you should consider yourself cured. Although there have been instances where melanoma cells have fooled pathologists, these instances are extremely rare. By far the greater risk is that you might develop a second primary melanoma. Careful observation of your remaining moles will help to ensure that any new lesions are caught before they become cancerous, or at least before the cancer has invaded deeply into the skin. If your primary melanoma was Clark's level II, your risk for internal recurrence of melanoma is small—10 to 15%. If you were diagnosed with Clark's level III or higher, there is a good chance that the melanoma cells may have spread, or metastasized, from the original site into the lymph and blood systems, even if they cannot be detected at the time of diagnosis.

Metastases are often classified as regional or systemic. *Regional metastases* are located in the first lymph node area draining the primary site and anywhere between the primary site and those lymph nodes. For example, one of our patients, Eliot, had a primary melanoma removed from the skin on his right calf. Four years later he was found to have nodules under the skin of his right upper leg and enlarged lymph nodes in his right groin that were proved by fine needle aspiration (FNA) to contain melanoma cells. We were unable to detect metastases anywhere else in his body, and his metastases were classified as regional. If Eliot is later found to have melanoma cells in his liver and lung, these new sites would be classified as *systemic metastases*. The terms that are used to describe these two conditions are *regionally advanced disease* and *advanced systemic disease*. Their treatment may be very different.

More about Metastases

Malignant melanoma is unique among cancers in that it will metastasize to almost any organ in the body; we do not know why. When most cancers spread, they like to grow in particular organs. For example, breast cancer cells usually spread to the bones, and colon cancer cells usually spread to the liver. Once melanoma cells are in the bloodstream, they pass through all the organs. To form a metastasis in an organ, melanoma cells must first adhere to a blood vessel in that organ. Then they must penetrate the wall of the blood vessel and set up a kind of nest in the tissue of the organ. Finally, they release cytokines that bring new blood vessels to them for nourishment. Once they have developed a blood supply of their own, they are off and growing.

Each organ has its own chemical environment. Most melanoma cells will find the environment of a particular organ hostile. They may be killed or they may simply not be able to perform one or more of the operations needed for tumor formation. As the melanoma cells mutate, however, one or more of them may become adapted to the environment of a particular organ and can begin to grow there.

Although melanoma cells may metastasize to any part of the body, metastases in the vast majority of melanoma patients do follow a pattern. They are most likely to show up first as subcutaneous (under the skin) nodules, or in the lymph nodes, and then in the lungs, liver, and brain. It is not unusual, however, to find that melanoma has metastasized to the spleen, adrenal glands, intestines, bones, or bone marrow. It is uncommon for melanoma to invade the heart, the muscles, or any of the remaining organs, but it is not unheard of. Patients who die of the disease are most likely to die of brain metastases, but by this time, they usually have tumors in many other parts of their bodies as well.

We will talk more about a brave melanoma patient named Franco in Chapter 12, but some of the things doctors learned as they vainly sought a treatment that would save Franco's life illustrate the complex nature of metastatic melanoma and the problems physicians and scientists must overcome in developing a cure or even effective treatments for the disease. Franco developed malignant melanoma as a teenager. Despite surgery and chemotherapy, the disease spread to nearly every organ in the boy's body as well as to his muscles and brain, and he eventually died. In an attempt to find a treatment to stop the spread of the disease, doctors took samples of melanoma from various of Franco's organs and analyzed them in the laboratory. The analysis showed that those cells that had proliferated in Franco's brain were very different from those in his liver or his lungs. In fact, each site had a characteristic population of melanoma cells that was different from all the others.

Melanoma often behaves this way when it metastasizes. And it is because melanoma mutates that it can invade so many parts of the body. This propensity to mutate is also an important reason why it is so difficult to develop drugs or vaccines that will attack all the melanoma cells in a person's body.

Scientists are working hard to figure out the mechanisms of melanoma metastases. Such understanding will be key to the development of new and better treatments. As we will see, the type of treatment currently used for metastatic melanoma depends on which organs are involved. Treatment may include chemotherapy, immunotherapy, surgery, radiation therapy, or a combination of these.

WILL TREATMENT HELP?

As we discuss the current treatments, we will frequently use the terms **partial remission** or **response** (PR), **complete remission** or **response** (CR), and **overall response rate.** Partial remission means that all the measurable metastases in a patient's body decrease in size by 50% or more in response to a given treatment. A complete remission is said to have occurred when physical examination, X rays, scans, and blood tests can no longer detect any signs of melanoma. The overall response rate for a specific treatment is based on the total number of patients having either a partial or a complete remission.

Complete remission does not necessarily mean permanent cure, unfortunately. It simply means that no melanoma can be found at a particular time by the available tests. Microscopic deposits of melanoma cells too small to be detected may still be lurking and can appear at a later time. In fact, this is likely to be true, because of that old problem—mutation. Although a given treatment may kill the majority of melanoma cells, some of the cells are probably resistant to the treatment. These resistant cells survive the treatment and are then free to proliferate but are usually too few to detect initially. Permanent cure of metastatic melanoma does occur, but to pronounce a patient cured requires many years of follow-up after treatment has ended. It is also never certain that the cure is due to the treatment: untreated patients sometimes experience remission and even cure.

"What are my chances?" This is a question that any doctor who has had to give a diagnosis of advanced melanoma has heard many times. Many variables help determine the outcome of any patient with metastatic melanoma, including the sites and extent of disease, the organs involved, the age and general health of the individual, the time from original diagnosis to development of metastases, the presence or absence of symptoms, and the site of the original melanoma. The number of variables makes predicting outcome in any single individual both difficult and hazardous. Each patient represents a unique situation for which statistics can only be used as a guideline.

If you have advanced melanoma, it is best to discuss *your situation* in detail with your physician, because the statistics that may apply in general may not be applicable to your particular case. What we say below, too, must be viewed carefully in the context and consideration of your own unique situation. Every physician who has cared for many melanoma patients has tales to tell about those who have defied all the odds.

With this in mind, here are the statistics: of those patients who develop metastases in regional lymph nodes draining the original primary site, 70–75% will eventually develop, or be found to have, other metastases in internal organs. Once melanoma is found in internal organs—that is, involvement of organs other than the skin or regional lymph nodes—life span is generally measured in months to a few years with an average of less than one year. For those who receive treatment and have a partial or complete remission (about 25%), the average survival is increased to an average of about 2 years, with some patients, perhaps 5%, experiencing permanent disappearance of the disease. The fewer the number of organs involved and the smaller the "bulk" of tumor burden, the better the prognosis. For people who develop brain metastases, survival averages 3–6 months from the time the brain metastases are discovered. An exception to this is the patient who develops only a single brain metastasis that can be removed surgically; though not common, this does happen occasionally.

These statistics are not pleasant to read, and we do not enjoy having to give them. We hope, however, that they will help patients with advanced melanoma and their families make the difficult decisions about what and how much treatment they want to receive for their disease and how they can spend the rest of their lives in the most comfortable and satisfying manner. The decision will be different for every patient. There are no right or wrong answers. We wish all melanoma patients could be cured.

TREATING REGIONAL LYMPH NODE RECURRENCE

As we have already learned, it is not uncommon for melanoma to appear in the regional lymph nodes months or years after the primary lesion was removed. This may occur in patients who did not have an elective regional lymph node dissection at the time of diagnosis, in patients who had this surgery but some of the lymph nodes were missed, or in patients who underwent elective regional lymph node dissection at a different site. Provided this is the only area where metastases are evident, the first treatment is complete removal of the lymph nodes in the involved area by a surgeon skilled in the procedure, usually a *surgical oncologist.* It is extremely important that *all* the lymph nodes in the area be removed. Partial removal of the lymph nodes—that is, attempting to find and remove only the lymph nodes containing melanoma—is virtually impossible, since small deposits of melanoma cannot be seen by the surgeon at the time of the operation. Such micrometastases can be detected only by dissecting the lymph nodes and looking at them under a microscope. (See the description of preparing a pathology sample in Chapter 7.)

If lymph nodes containing melanoma are inadvertently left behind, the cancer cells in them often begin to grow more rapidly than before. This results in new tumors in the same place, requiring more surgery that is very difficult due to the scar tissue left behind from the original operation. We do not know why melanoma cell growth is stimulated in an area where surgery has recently been performed, but it is a well-recognized and dreaded problem in melanoma treatment. The most likely explanation is that growth factors or cytokines released locally to facilitate wound healing also stimulate the melanoma cells. Regardless of the reason, we strongly advise complete removal of all the lymph nodes in the region.

To date, chemotherapy before or after the surgery has not been shown to be beneficial, but this is an area of continued investigation. In some cases, your physician may advise local radiation therapy following surgery (see Chapter 9). As we noted above, alpha interferon has also been used at this point, but given the recent large study calling the benefit of interferon into question, we no longer recommend it.

In Transit Metastases

In transit metastases is the name given to recurrences, usually seen as lumps in or under the skin, that develop between the primary site and the regional lymph nodes. This problem is seen most commonly on the legs in patients who have already had their regional lymph nodes removed. A typical example is David, a 40-year-old lawyer who had a primary melanoma removed from the right calf and at the time of the original diagnosis had an elective regional lymph node dissection of the right groin. Four years later, David returned to the doctor with multiple black lumps or nodules under the skin extending from the primary site to the upper leg. Almost always there are many more smaller deposits that cannot be seen or felt initially.

If there are only a few nodules, they can be removed surgically, but more are likely to appear with time. If there are numerous nodules, more drastic measures may be needed. The most commonly used procedure is called **regional limb perfusion.** In this procedure the blood vessels supplying the leg involved are isolated and high doses of chemotherapy drugs or cytokines are pumped through the leg, sometimes with simultaneous heating of the limb, called **hyperthermia.** A variety of chemotherapy drugs, especially one called melphalan, may temporarily control the problem. More recently, doctors have begun using the cytokines gamma interferon and tumor necrosis factor alpha (TNF), both alone and in combination with melphalan. They have reported higher success rates using this combination, but the test groups so far are small. Neither surgery nor regional limb perfusion affects the likelihood of the disease recurring in different sites.

TREATING SYSTEMIC METASTASES

The treatment of melanoma that has spread to the internal organs is constantly undergoing change. Currently there is no single best treatment for all patients. The type of treatment offered to a patient with systemic metastases depends on many factors, including where the metastases are, how many organs are involved, what problems they are causing, and the general health of the patient. Your physician should be familiar with the current research studies available and should use the results of these studies to assess the likelihood that the treatment she or he proposes will be helpful and not harmful to you. Because of these variables and the rapid changes taking place in therapy, we cannot make specific recommendations for individual patients. Instead, we will give a broad outline of the treatments currently in use and suggest some of the issues you may want to think about in making a decision about whether or not to undergo the treatment. In Chapter 13, we will discuss some of the new treatments being investigated in research studies.

Single Drugs Used to Treat Metastatic Melanoma

When a patient is diagnosed with one systemic metastasis, the presumption is that there are probably many more, even though they may not be detectable at the time. Occasionally a person will be lucky enough to have only a single metastasis that may be removed surgi-

| *An encouraging word about chemotherapy* | Everyone has heard horror stories about chemotherapy. Most of the bad rap was about the disabling nausea and vomiting that patients experienced. Fortunately, there are new and effective anti-nausea medications that can eliminate or nearly eliminate nausea in almost all patients with few or no side effects. These drugs can be given intravenously and also come in pill form. The first and still the most popular one is ondansetron (Zofran), but as so often happens, newer cousins have been released. Chemotherapy nowadays is often so well tolerated that many patients continue to work during treatments. |

cally and result in cure, but this is unusual. Almost all patients with systemic metastases will require treatment that will travel throughout the entire body, such as chemotherapy or immunotherapy.

DTIC (DACARBAZINE)

DTIC is the chemotherapy drug most commonly used to treat metastatic melanoma. It has been used for melanoma patients since the late 1960s, and no other single drug has yet been shown to be as effective. Despite the drug's long use, doctors and researchers still don't fully understand how it fights melanoma. We know that, like most other chemotherapy drugs, it acts by randomly killing cells that are dividing more rapidly than normal, but this is not the whole story, since there are many other drugs with similar cell-killing power that have little or no effect on melanoma.

DTIC is usually given as a short intravenous infusion in an office or clinic 3–5 days in a row; the series of infusions is repeated every 3 weeks. The major side effects are severe nausea, muscle aches, and lowering of the blood cell counts. The nausea can usually be easily controlled by the use of the anti-nausea medications described on p. 128 ("An encouraging word about chemotherapy"). Hair loss (alopecia), the side effect of chemotherapy that patients often dread most, is minimal.

Unfortunately, the benefit is limited. Only 20–25% of patients will achieve a partial or complete regression of their melanoma. As with all other treatments we will discuss, responses are seen most often in those with disease limited to the skin, lymph nodes, or lung, although regression in other sites is sometimes seen. DTIC is not effective against brain metastases because the drug cannot penetrate the barrier that keeps most of the substances in the bloodstream out of the brain.

TEMAZOLAMIDE (TEMADOL)

Temazolamide is a drug recently introduced for the treatment of metastatic melanoma. Chemically, it is a cousin of DTIC, and it probably works in a similar way. Its advantage is that it can be given either intravenously or by mouth. It may also provide some benefit to patients with brain metastases. Laboratory studies have shown that, unlike many other chemotherapy drugs, temazolamide penetrates into the brain. Physicians and researchers hope that temazolamide may help shrink brain metastases, particularly when they are small, but its effectiveness on brain tumors has yet to be proven in a large human study.

The current practice is to give the drug in pill form for 3 weeks, followed by 1 week off, and to repeat the cycle every 4 weeks. To optimize the amount of drug taken up by the body, patients should take it in the morning on an empty stomach. The side effects are similar to those seen with DTIC, with nausea and lowering of the blood counts being most common. Hair loss is rare. The overall response rate to temazolamide has been about 20%. As with DTIC, patients with melanoma in their lungs, lymph nodes, and skin usually have the best response.

FOTEMUSTINE

Fotemustine is another relatively new chemotherapy drug used in the treatment of metastatic melanoma. It has been studied extensively in Europe, particularly in France. It belongs to a class of chemotherapy drugs called the nitrosoureas (other drugs in this class are CCNU and BCNU). Like temazolamide, these drugs have been shown to penetrate well into the brain. Fotemustine is usually given as a short intravenous infusion once weekly for 4 weeks. The major side effect is a lowering of the white blood cell count. Hair loss is also common, but nausea is mild if it occurs at all. The overall response rate is about 20%—similar to that seen with DTIC and temazolamide— but some well-documented cases of regression of brain metastases have also been reported. Currently, fotemustine has been approved for use only in Europe, but it can usually be obtained through your oncologist or cancer center in the United States.

ALPHA INTERFERON

If you have read Chapter 9 on adjuvant therapy, you will already be acquainted with alpha interferon. It is one of the many cytokines that have been tested in melanoma and the one with which physicians have had the greatest experience. How alpha interferon works is not completely understood, but we know that it works very differently from any of the chemotherapy drugs discussed above.

Alpha interferon, like all cytokines, is produced naturally by the body. It does not act by directly killing cancer or melanoma cells, like chemotherapy drugs do. Instead, it stimulates the cells of the immune system to do the actual killing, while at the same time making the cancer cells easier for the immune system to detect.

Alpha interferon can be given either by intravenous or by subcutaneous injection. It is given in doses that are much greater than those made naturally by the body. Doctors usually teach patients how to self-administer the drug by injecting it under their skin, usually three times per week. These are similar to the injections that many people with diabetes use to self-administer insulin one or more times a day. Most patients can learn to give themselves injections without difficulty, but some prefer to have a family member or friend give them.

With the first few injections almost everyone has a flu-like reaction, with shaking chills, fever, and muscle aches. This usually diminishes after a few weeks of treatment, but many patients are left with a feeling of chronic tiredness as long as the treatment continues, particularly if high doses are used. Most patients take their injections at bedtime so they sleep through most of the side effects. Tylenol or aspirin is often prescribed before the injection to reduce any fever that may occur.

People taking interferon have reported a whole host of other side effects, but the most common include weight loss, mild hair loss, depression, and loss of libido (sex drive). Also common are lowering of blood cell counts and elevation of the liver blood tests. One peculiar side effect is severe worsening of psoriasis in patients who already suffer from this skin disorder; this is often so bad that the interferon treatment must be discontinued.

Like almost every other drug used alone to treat melanoma, the overall response rate is around 20%. Again, these responses are usually seen in patients with disease confined to the skin, lymph nodes, and lungs. Some patients, however, have had long-term remissions (as long as 10 years after treatments were stopped), and they may well be cured. This rare long-term benefit has also occurred with such other treatments as interleukin 2 and monoclonal antibodies. Alpha interferon has no apparent benefit in the treatment of brain metastases.

IL-2 was heralded as a possible miracle cure for melanoma when it was first introduced and tested in the 1980s. Unfortunately, it did not live up to this billing, and we now have more realistic expectations of its effectiveness. IL-2 is a cytokine similar to interferon, but with a somewhat different effect on the cells of the immune system. Like interferon, it can be given intravenously or in subcutaneous injections, but the intravenous method is currently favored. When given by vein, it is run continuously through an IV over several days in a hospital setting while the patient is monitored closely to prevent serious side effects such as kidney damage or a marked fall in blood pressure. At most medical centers, dopamine, a medication that raises the blood pressure, is given throughout the IL-2 infusion. Other side effects may include muscle aches and pains and fatigue. The response rate to IL-2 alone is less than 20%, and it is now used almost exclusively in conjunction with other drugs, as described later in this chapter. As with alpha interferon, however, some patients taking IL-2 have experienced complete prolonged remissions. Like alpha interferon, IL-2 has no effect on brain metastases.

other drugs

Virtually every cancer chemotherapy drug ever discovered has been tried in patients with advanced melanoma. Some—including velban, cisplatinum, BCNU, and vincristine—have had response rates of around 10% when given alone, but none of them has been shown to be of consistent long-term benefit. Their use instead has been primarily in multidrug treatment regimens such as those discussed below.

Multidrug Therapy of Metastatic Melanoma

The use of multiple drugs with different mechanisms of action has become routine in the treatment of most cancers, and melanoma is no exception. Cancer drugs kill cells in many different ways. Some act by interfering with cell metabolism, others cause damage to the DNA in the cells (mortally wounding them), and still others interfere with the process of cell division. Others, such as tamoxifen (discussed below), have effects in melanoma that are not understood. The cy-tokines, by contrast, arm the immune system to do the killing.

The object with a multidrug approach is to combine all of these to attack the cancer cells on many different fronts. The drugs that are selected for a program are usually those that have shown some bene-fit when they were tested alone in melanoma. Thus, you will see DTIC in almost every multidrug regimen because it is still the best single drug for the treatment of metastatic melanoma.

An attempt is made to select a combination of drugs that do not have the same toxicities or side effects. This is not always possible, par-ticularly when it comes to suppression of the blood cell counts. For this reason, these drug combinations are usually given in high doses for a few days every 3–4 weeks. The rest periods in between are to al-low the blood cell counts to return to normal or near normal before the next course is given. Sometimes the dose of one or more drugs may need to be reduced.

A large number of different combinations of drugs have been or are being tested in melanoma. There are too many to mention here, and each has its advocates. For the moment, no single program can be said to be vastly superior to any other program and none has satis-factorily been able to deal with the problem of brain metastases.

THE DARTMOUTH REGIMEN

This is probably the most commonly used multidrug program currently in use. It combines the chemotherapy drugs DTIC, cisplat-inum, and BCNU with a commonly used breast cancer pill called ta-moxifen (Nolvadex). Tamoxifen is used to treat breast cancer because of its anti-estrogen effect. It was originally added to a melanoma treat-ment program because it was thought that some melanoma cells might also be feeding on estrogens produced in the body. It has since become clear, however, that tamoxifen works through some other mechanism in melanoma; exactly how has not yet been determined. BCNU was added in the hope that it might be beneficial against brain involvement since, like its cousin fotemustine, it is able to penetrate the blood-brain barrier.

The three chemotherapy drugs are given by vein every 3–4 weeks, usually in an outpatient setting. Tamoxifen tablets are taken daily by mouth. There are many variations on this program, but the side effects and results are similar with all of them, namely, a 30–35% overall response rate. Ten percent of patients have a complete remission, and 20–25% have a partial remission. Suppression of the blood counts is the major toxicity, and recurrence of melanoma in the brain is common even with complete remission in other organs.

COMBINATIONS OF CHEMOTHERAPY AND CYTOKINES

A variety of combinations of chemotherapy drugs with alpha interferon and/or IL-2 are currently being tested in centers around the world. Almost all include the chemotherapy drugs DTIC and cisplatinum; some also add velban and/or BCNU. In the most rigorous combination, all of these are used along with both IL-2 and alpha interferon. Although the toxicity of these rigorous programs is high, the reported overall response rates in small initial trials are above 50%. This treatment is currently in the experimental stage and is restricted primarily to large melanoma treatment centers. The benefit for prevention of brain metastases remains to be determined.

One note of caution: All the chemotherapy drugs used in melanoma, including those with demonstrated benefits in shrinking metastases, suppress the immune system. This suppression is usually short-lived, but it is a real and important factor in cancer treatment. No one has yet devised a chemotherapy drug that can simultaneously kill cancer cells and enhance the immune response against them. One of the aims of adding cytokines to chemotherapy is to deal with this problem, but the effect is never complete. If you are receiving chemotherapy, you should discuss with your doctor how severe the effects of the specific drugs you are taking might be on your immune system and blood cells and what precautions you should take to avoid infection.

SURGICAL REMOVAL OF METASTASES

Surgery is often the recommended treatment for brain metastases (we will discuss this below). There are many instances, however, where surgical removal of metastases in areas other than the brain may also be the best treatment, even when the melanoma has invaded many organs. This is true for troublesome metastases that have not responded to other treatments, are causing pain or other symptoms, and can be removed without damaging normal organ function or other serious consequences. Examples of this are metastases in the intestine that are continually bleeding, metastases in the spleen (located in the left upper abdomen) that cause discomfort and a sensation of fullness after only a few bites of food, painful metastases in muscles, and metastases in the heart that cause the heart to fail or to beat abnormally.

Another instance where surgery may be a good choice is when a patient is left with one or two metastases after drug therapy has led to remission in all other areas. The assumption is made that these residual deposits of melanoma contain clones of cells resistant to the drug treatments and that their removal may prevent further spread. The number of patients for whom such treatment would be considered is small, however, and no studies have been done to test its effectiveness.

THE TREATMENT OF BRAIN METASTASES

Of all the body's organs, the brain is the organ in which melanoma is most likely to metastasize. Despite advances in treating metastases outside the brain, no consistently effective treatment has been found for brain metastases, either to prevent them or to treat them effectively when they occur.

Melanocytes, the cells that give rise to melanoma, actually start their life in the embryo as a part of the developing nervous system, of which the brain is a major part. This is probably why melanoma cells seem to find, in the brain, a compatible place in which to grow and prosper. Melanoma cells travel to the brain through the bloodstream and settle down to feed and grow like little ticking time bombs. Seventy percent or more of patients with metastatic melanoma will develop brain metastases. Sometimes melanoma will spread first to the brain, but more commonly it spreads to other organs first.

Symptoms of brain metastases depend on where the tumors are located. Some parts of the brain are less important than others, and big tumors can grow there for a time with little consequence. Other areas of the brain are critical for movement, feeling, speech, vision, or even consciousness; and even small tumors in these locations can cause severe problems. The most common symptoms of brain metastases are persistent headaches, seizures, dizziness, drowsiness, or numbness or weakness in one or more limbs.

Brain metastases are the most common cause of death in melanoma patients, because as the tumors grow, they eventually crush and kill normal brain tissue that is necessary for life. The average period of survival of a melanoma patient with brain metastases who receives no treatment is 3–6 months from the time the brain metastases are first discovered. Treatment, and the outcome after treatment, both depend on how many areas of the brain are involved, which areas of the brain are involved, and the presence or absence of metastases elsewhere in the body.

Surgical Removal of Brain Metastases

Recent years have seen rapid advances both in brain imaging (MRI and CT scans) and in neurosurgical techniques. With these advances has come the ability to remove some melanoma brain metastases without great difficulty, and frequently with survival benefit. People who should be considered for surgical treatment of brain metastases are those with a limited number of metastases (three or fewer) which are located in areas that can be reached by the surgeon without causing damage to the normal brain. People who have multiple metastases, one or two of which are immediately life threatening or causing problems, may also sometimes be treated with surgery if the tumors in question are surgically accessible.

Surgery is rarely curative, because other metastases usually appear with time, but it often provides improved quality of life and prevents or postpones some of the devastating consequences of brain metastases, such as paralysis, blindness, or loss of speech. Surprisingly, this surgery is usually very well tolerated, and many patients can be released from the hospital only a few days after surgery.

Standard Radiation Therapy for Brain Metastases

You may have noticed that we have not yet mentioned radiation treatment in any detail. That is because melanoma, unlike many other types of cancer, is not very sensitive to radiation. The use of radiation is generally limited to the brain and troublesome recurrences in the lymph nodes, especially after one or more surgeries have already been undertaken in the area. Radiation has been the primary method of treatment of brain metastases for many years and is used for patients with many areas of the brain involved and for lesions that are not accessible to the surgeon.

Usually the whole brain is treated using a radiation therapy machine called a *linear accelerator*. The patient lies on a special table, and powerful X rays are shot through the brain like tiny bullets. The idea is not only to treat the areas that can be seen on the brain scan, but to eliminate smaller deposits of melanoma that are not visible. The treatments are usually given daily for 5–21 days. The most common side effects are nausea and hair loss, which is usually complete but reversible. Patients who have multiple metastases should consider whole brain radiation, but only with the understanding that it is of limited benefit in most cases. About half of the patients who have this treatment experience partial remission. On average this prolongs life for about three months.

The Gamma Knife and Stereotactic Radiosurgery for Brain Metastases

The **gamma knife** and **stereotactic radiosurgery** are two new ways of delivering focused radiation to specific lesions or areas of the brain. The methods used to deliver the radiation in these two techniques are somewhat different from each other, but the objectives and results are similar. In both techniques several powerful beams of radiation coming from different angles around the head focus on a specific part of the brain. This eliminates some of the radiation going to normal brain tissue and allows much larger doses to be delivered directly to the metastases.

The gamma knife and stereotactic radiosurgery are used only in patients who have lesions in only a few areas of the brain. The techniques may be particularly useful for treating metastases that are deep in the brain where surgical removal is impossible. Initial reports suggest that this type of radiation treatment is effective but is useful only when there are few metastases and they are small (2 centimeters or less). These forms of treatment are now available in most large medical centers.

Drugs for the Treatment of Brain Metastases

Unfortunately, most chemotherapy drugs and cytokines penetrate poorly into the brain. As a result, very few of them have any effect on brain metastases. Fotemustine and temazolamide, two drugs that have had limited success, are discussed above. Their overall and long-term benefit remains to be determined.

Drugs can relieve some of the symptoms of melanoma of the brain, however, and thus improve the quality of the patient's life. When melanoma metastases develop in the brain, the body reacts by producing fluid, or swelling, around them. This is called *edema* and can be seen on the brain scan as a black, clear area around the melanoma. This is similar to the swelling that occurs when you twist your ankle or break your wrist. The edema that develops after an ankle injury, however, just pushes out against the skin. The brain is in a closed, inelastic space (the skull), and the swelling may cause problems by pushing and cramping the brain against the skull bone. This in itself may cause many of the early problems patients with brain metastases report, particularly headache. The edema can usually be easily relieved by the administration of a cortisone (steroid)-like drug called dexamethasone (decadron). Most patients with brain metastases need decadron at one time or another, and it may be required for many months. It has no anticancer effect but is used solely to relieve the pressure caused by the swelling.

Similarly, many patients with brain metastases require the drug phenytoin (Dilantin) to prevent seizures that are often caused by the brain metastases. Dilantin has no anticancer effect, either, and is used only to improve quality of life by suppressing seizures. Your doctor must monitor blood levels of Dilantin carefully to make sure the proper dose of the medication is given. Too little will not prevent seizures, and too much will cause side effects such as confusion or unsteadiness.

NEW AND EXPERIMENTAL TREATMENTS

The treatments discussed above are all being used by melanoma specialists today. You may have heard or read about numerous other treatments for melanoma that are not mentioned here, including monoclonal antibody therapy, gene therapy, and anti-angiogenesis agents. These and other experimental therapies are discussed in Chapter 13, which covers ongoing research in the field.

ALTERNATIVE TREATMENTS

This subject alone would require another whole book. The list of alternative treatments is almost endless and includes diets of various kinds, vitamins, blue-green algae, melatonin, laetrile, enemas, liver cleansing, starvation diets, crystals, selenium, zinc, aroma therapy, and many more. Almost every patient with metastatic melanoma will try one form or another of these therapies on the advice of family and well-meaning friends. Most do no harm unless used in excess, and many, such as meditation and a healthy diet, may improve the general well-being of the patient; but the benefit of these therapies in treating melanoma has not been proven using the same rigorous scientific techniques that are required of standard cancer treatments. Most doctors would neither encourage nor discourage their use in moderation, but it is important to discuss the use of any such treatments openly with your health care providers.

Another word of caution: Patients with advanced melanoma and their families are often understandably clutching at straws in their attempts to find effective treatment. There are charlatans out there who prey on this vulnerability. Beware of expensive therapies or unknown chemicals touted by individuals who have no medical credentials. The results of these scams can be tragic for both patients and families.

Doctors also worry about patients' spending time, energy, and money on unproven therapies—and, as a consequence, avoiding or not keeping up with treatment that has been proven to help. Most doctors will advise you about which *complementary therapies* can hurt, which might help, and which may not help but, in any case, will do no harm. Complementary therapies are nonmedical therapies such as relaxation therapy, homeopathy, acupuncture, herbal remedies, and magnet therapy.

Advanced malignant melanoma is a terrible emotional burden as well as a debilitating physical disease. Patients' reactions vary. Some insist on trying any treatment, no matter how uncomfortable it may make them or how slim the chances of its success. Others refuse any treatment at all, preferring to spend the time they have left in places other than a doctor's office or a hospital. Most fall somewhere between these extremes.

Physicians, too, may differ in their approach because each patient has his or her own unique characteristics and because so few treatments have been fully tested that there are no maps showing the road to remission. Some doctors will be more aggressive in recommending treatment than others. Often, they can only fall back on their experience and that of their colleagues, recommending a particular therapy because it seemed to provide some benefit to previous patients.

Whatever course of treatment patient and doctor agree upon, however, there is no need for the patient to suffer great physical pain. In the next chapter we will talk about treating pain and about patients' options when it is time to stop treating the disease.

· · ·

11

Managing Pain and the End of Life

W hatever the limits of medical science in providing treatments to cure advanced melanoma, there is a great deal a
physician can do to alleviate the pain that may accom-
pany the disease. When a person with melanoma has decided not to
pursue further treatment or the doctor has had to break the bad news
that there are no more effective treatments available, expectations
may change. The physician may take on a new role—that of *caring*
rather than *curing*. Physicians have become much better, and more
comfortable, in that role in recent years.

There is no set time when pain will occur (if it occurs at all). It
depends on where the cancer is. Metastases in the bones and spinal
cord area are usually very painful, for example, while those in the lung
don't hurt, although they do cause shortness of breath. Some people
have little pain during the course of the disease, even up until the time
of death, while for others pain is constant and progressive, requiring
constant and progressive treatment.

The mainstay of pain control is morphine. Long-acting morphine tablets that come in various strengths are now available. They
release the morphine slowly, over 12 hours, so the patient does not
have to get up at night to take a dose and can go out to dinner or the
movies without fear that pain will interrupt a pleasant evening.
The dose can be increased as needed without any real upper limit. The
usual starting dose is 30 milligrams twice per day, but we have treated
patients with as much as 3,000 milligrams per day when necessary.
The major side effects of morphine are drowsiness (which becomes
less of a problem with time), constipation (a real problem that has to
be treated from the start), and nausea (which also usually clears up

fairly quickly or can be controlled with medication). After a few days of taking morphine tablets, a person should be able to function normally, but we advise against driving or doing other activities where safety depends on optimum alertness. Quick-acting liquid morphine is available and is freely used to treat pain that breaks through the long-acting doses. (Called *breakthrough pain,* this is pain that occurs prior to the next regularly scheduled long-acting dose.)

For those who cannot take morphine because of nausea or constipation, newer, long-acting pain medications such as Fentanyl are available. These are administered by applying a "patch" loaded with the medication to the skin. The medication is released slowly, over three days, and is absorbed through the skin. The side effects of these drugs are similar to those of morphine, but they cause less constipation. These drugs are also much more expensive than morphine, which costs very little.

Finally, to treat severe pain, a number of drugs can be delivered continuously, either intravenously or under the skin. Again, the most common is morphine, which frequently is administered through a small needle inserted under the skin. The needle is attached to a small pump (about the size of a beeper) containing the morphine which delivers the morphine at a slow and constant rate. These devices also have a button that the patient can push to get a booster dose if there is breakthrough pain. These drugs are used in conjunction with other pain medications such as the nonsteroidal anti-inflammatories, or NSAIDs (ibuprofen, naprosyn, clinoril, etc.), Tylenol, and often some kind of sedation medication or muscle relaxant such as Valium.

Although not all melanoma patients experience physical pain, most suffer from emotional distress. The frightening nature of the disease, and the uncertainty about its course, are terribly upsetting. Most large cancer centers have melanoma support groups. These usually include patients with all stages of the disease. A social worker, nurse, or physician attends these meetings and acts as an advisor. Doctors commonly prescribe antidepressants in cases of advanced melanoma. Some are useful in augmenting pain relief as well as in helping to reduce depression. Developing a regimen of drugs which will keep the patient as physically and emotionally comfortable as possible is a primary objective of treatment in late-stage melanoma.

The Physician's Point of View

One of the most difficult times for any physician is when she or he has to explain to a patient that there is no therapy left that will effectively treat a disease such as metastatic melanoma. "I can't do any more for you" are the most painful words a doctor can say—for the patient, for the family, and for the doctor.

The whole of a physician's training is geared to curing. When that cannot be done, doctors often experience the lack of ability to cure as a personal failure. At the same time, doctors always experience a tremendous feeling of frustration that they can't do more. Where are all those miracle cures that the papers talk about? Why can't the scientists move faster? Will we ever be able to cure this disease? All these questions run through a doctor's mind when he or she finally has to face the fact that everything has been tried but nothing has worked. There is no instruction in medical school on how to break this news to the patient and deal with your own feelings of sadness and frustration and failure. All of us handle it in our own way, and it is not always satisfactory. The best that can be said is that it often leads to a renewed desire to try to find new answers and solutions.

Taking Care of the Whole Patient

For people with metastatic disease who choose not to have treatment and people whose disease progresses despite treatment, there has been a dramatic and enlightened change in the services and therapies available to make the process of dying more comfortable and dignified. Most cancer centers have what are called palliative care programs to do just this. Often available 24 hours a day, they provide counseling to patients and family members about what to expect and how to manage symptoms such as pain and nausea. They also provide information about home and **hospice** care. For people who choose to stay at home for their remaining days, home hospice services are now available in most cities. In consultation with a doctor or a palliative care service, they provide medical, psychological, and spiritual support in the home for the patient and the family. For those who cannot be cared for at home, in-patient hospices are also widely available.

A LOOK AT HOSPICES

In the past, many people viewed hospices as sad, grim places to go and die. Today, nothing could be further from the truth. Hospices are havens where a person can go to live out his or her remaining time in peace and comfort. The objective of hospice programs is to make the remaining time as comfortable and enjoyable as possible. The concept of hospice is not new, but the hospice movement has gained new popularity and well-deserved recognition around the world in recent years. Hospices are now a regular and important part of cancer care.

There are two kinds of hospice care, in-patient and home hospice. Deciding which of these is best depends upon individual circumstances, and the use of home hospice services does not preclude using in-patient hospice, and vice versa. Both kinds of hospices are covered by most insurance programs and HMOs. For people without insurance coverage who cannot afford the customary charges, hospices can usually provide their services at a reduced rate that is tailored to the patient's financial situation. Home hospice support is often a good option when the patient's needs are limited and there are adequate caregivers available in the home. All of the pain-relieving medications and other medications that may be required can usually be given in the home. Home hospice services are staffed by qualified palliative care nurses and physicians and often include volunteer members who have been through a similar process with a loved one, bringing a measure of experience and knowledge that is both comforting and reassuring.

When 24-hour care is needed, or when no one is available in the home, an in-patient hospice is usually the best option. It relieves family and friends of what can be very intensive caregiving, so they can spend all of their available time enjoying the company of their loved one. In-patient hospices are available in most cities, often in quiet locations. Their atmosphere is homelike, giving a serene feeling of love and care, and they have open visiting hours for family and friends. They are staffed by dedicated personnel, including specialized physicians and counselors. The patient's personal physician is also usually involved in making decisions and providing care.

Both types of hospices deal effectively and kindly with the major fears that most dying people have—fears of severe unrelenting pain, loss of dignity, and loss of control. The new pain-delivery methods described above ensure that most patients can now experience a relatively pain-free end to life. Importantly, this can almost always be done without the patient's suffering undue drowsiness or loss of mental faculties. Dignity and control are preserved. Patients can take care of unfinished business and visit with family and friends.

Death will eventually come to all of us, but all too often we do not have the option of choosing the place or circumstances. It may be of little comfort to say that if you have metastatic melanoma you may have that option. Although we encourage optimism and a "positive outlook," the time may well come when the best option is a dignified and comfortable death in a place of your choosing.

Mark's Story

Mark was a 44-year-old physician in a small town with a busy practice and healthy lifestyle. He always thought of himself as a strong and independent man. He took care of other people— they didn't need to take care of him. He hiked alone in rugged mountains, skydived, and was always available to his wife, his two teenage children, and his patients.

When Mark was 39 he had a deep Clark's level 4 melanoma removed from his back. He had no further problems until just before his 44th birthday, when he developed a cough, fatigue, and headaches that would not go away. A CT scan showed that the melanoma had spread to multiple sites in his brain, lungs, and bone. He vowed to fight the disease to the end, and he visited major melanoma centers around the United States seeking a cure. Eventually he was treated with a combination of chemotherapy and radiation therapy. Although he improved slightly for a few weeks, he then began to have severe, unrelenting pain in his hips and back, where the melanoma was growing at a rapid rate. Being a physician, he tried to medicate himself and was determined that he would get better, but the pain only grew worse until he could no longer sleep or sit for more than a few minutes. He was miserable, angry, and exhausted, and his wife and children were at their wits' end as to how to deal with him.

When the pain became too great, Mark finally agreed to be admitted to a hospital where he was seen by the palliative care team. They gave him intravenous morphine, and in just a few hours his pain was tolerable. In a few days, it was all but gone. Doctors then substituted long-acting oral morphine tablets along with an antidepressant, and Mark was discharged a few days later. With his pain under control, Mark was able to regain his independence and sense of humor. He had come to the understanding that time was limited and precious, and he wanted to live it the best and most comfortable way possible—to enjoy his last days in peace and comfort with his family. He closed his practice and walked in the mountains with his family and even caught a trout in his favorite fishing hole. His strength, however, was waning with each day, and he knew that he and his wife would need help before the end came.

Mark's town had both in-patient and home hospice care. The home hospice was the option Mark and his family chose. The team, consisting of a doctor, nurses, and volunteers, visited and helped arrange their house so that Mark had a bed and a big comfortable chair in the living room where he could look out over the mountains he loved. Members of the team came daily and helped Mark adjust his pain medication. When he was no longer able to swallow tablets, they provided an infusion set that he and his wife could regulate to keep him comfortable. When he could no longer stand to urinate, they provided a catheter for his bladder. They arranged for someone to come to the house when his wife needed to shop or visit friends, and they were available by telephone 24 hours a day, which was a great comfort to all.

Thanks to the hospice, Mark died comfortably at home in his chair looking out at the mountains with his family by his side. There were no heart monitors or wires or tubes down his throat—just peace and comfort and love for a strong and independent man.

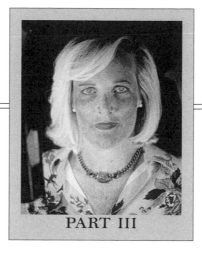

PART III

MELANOMA
Less Common Types and Melanoma Research

Fair-skinned, Caucasian adults are most
likely to develop melanoma, but people of all
races can develop the disease, and more and
more children are being diagnosed with
melanoma, as well. Laboratory research and
clinical research are exploring promising
new therapies for the treatment
of melanoma.

12

Unusual Forms of Melanoma

U p to this point we have described melanomas that begin with a spot on the skin that, if not caught soon enough, can metastasize throughout the body. These are by far the most common melanomas, and most of them occur in Caucasians. As we explained in the opening chapters of this book, however, melanoma can strike anyone; and it can begin wherever melanocytes are found: eyes, rectum, vagina, intestines, mouth and gums, palms and soles of the feet, under fingernails and toenails, and even in the covering of the brain and spinal cord. Melanoma can begin in all of these sites; fortunately, it does so only rarely.

Like the melanocytes in the skin, melanocytes in the eyes produce melanin pigments to protect neighboring cells from the harmful effects of the sun. Melanin cells in other parts of the body presumably serve another function, since most of these other areas are never exposed to the sun and therefore do not need the sun-protecting properties of melanin. Melanins (there are several types) are remarkable pigments that are present in one form or another in almost all living things, including animals, plants, and microorganisms. In addition to protecting cells from the damaging effects of the sun's UV light, they also have the ability to detoxify many potentially dangerous substances. This is probably their function in non-skin locations.

Because the melanocytes in these areas are not exposed to the sun (sun exposure, of course, is the major cause of melanoma that begins in the skin), there must be other reasons that these cells become cancerous. What these reasons are, we do not yet know. In this chapter, we will discuss what we know about these noncutaneous melanomas as well as what's different about melanoma occurring in special patient populations.

NONCUTANEOUS FORMS OF MELANOMA

Melanoma with Unknown Primary Site

In about 5% of all melanoma cases, the first evidence that a person has the disease will be when doctors find a tumor in the person's lymph nodes or in one or more internal organs. When a biopsy of this tumor is examined microscopically, it is found to contain melanoma cells. The physician's first instinct will probably be to look over every nook and cranny of the skin, including between the toes, behind the ears, and on the scalp, for evidence of abnormal moles that might be melanoma. The doctor will also question the patient about any moles that he or she may have had removed in the past or any that have disappeared on their own. It is possible that melanoma cells fooled the original pathologist, but such cases are rare.

Usually there is no history of prior mole removal, and the doctor finds no abnormal moles on the patient's body. Then the logical question is, "Where did the internal melanoma come from if there isn't a melanoma on the skin?" This is a very good question because, as we have seen, melanocytes normally exist in many places in the body, but they are not normally found in the lymph nodes, in bone, or in lung, liver, or other internal organs. The presumption in such cases is that the person did have a melanoma on the skin at one time, but that it was attacked by the immune system and disappeared before it was even recognized by the patient, but not before it spread into the bloodstream or lymphatic channels in the deeper layers of the skin. Occasionally a patient will recall having had a mole months or years earlier that bled and "fell off," supporting this notion.

Sometimes patients become concerned when the primary lesion cannot be found. In truth, though, it makes little difference in outcome. Melanoma in the lung, for example, is melanoma in the lung, regardless of where the primary lesion, if any, was located. Stage for stage, there is no difference in outcome for patients with undiagnosed primaries compared to those with a known primary. Treatment and

management proceed just as they would if the cancer had metastasized from a known primary.

Melanoma of the Eye (Ocular Melanoma)

Melanocytes are found normally in many parts of the eye, including the back of the eye (the retina), the colored part of the eye (the
iris), and the pink inside lining of the eyelids (the conjunctiva). Nevi
may arise on and in the eye, but the percentage of eye nevi that
become melanoma is extremely small. The most common site for
melanoma is the back of the eye, where melanocytes are most plenti-
ful. **Ocular melanoma** may also arise, however, without a known
preexisting mole. No one knows what causes melanoma to develop in
the eye, but exposure to the sun is probably a factor. Indeed, the highest incidence of ocular melanoma is in fair-skinned Caucasians,
particularly persons with light eye colors such as blue, gray, or green.
People with the atypical mole syndrome have an increased likelihood
of having moles in the back of their eyes and so have an increased risk
of developing ocular melanoma, just as they do of developing cutaneous melanoma. For this reason, all patients with the atypical mole
syndrome should have a yearly examination of the back of the eye by
an ophthalmologist.

As you might guess, the diagnosis of ocular melanoma is often
delayed because the developing tumor is not easily noticed as it would
be on the skin. Further, it is not always easy to distinguish between a
benign mole and an early melanoma by examination of the eye, even
by the most highly trained specialist. Biopsy, so easily performed on
skin lesions, usually cannot be done on ocular moles for fear of permanent damage to the eye. Specialized tests including ultrasound and
MRI scans and a dye test called *fluorescein angiography* are useful,
but they may have to be repeated at frequent intervals to determine
if the lesion is growing. An enlarging pigmented lesion is likely to be
malignant, whereas one that does not change is probably a benign
mole. Advanced lesions often result in partial vision loss, bleeding into
the eye, or detachment of the retina, symptoms that lead to evaluation and subsequent diagnosis.

Small melanomas in the eye can be treated with laser therapy that allows vision to be preserved in about two-thirds of cases. In this treatment, special dyes are injected into the bloodstream. They are taken up by the cancer cells and sensitize them to the effects of the laser beams. Large melanomas, however, are best treated by complete surgical removal of the eye in an operation called *enucleation*. The patient can later be fitted with an artificial eye, which is manufactured to match the remaining eye and appears very realistic. The best treatment for medium-sized melanomas of the eye has not been determined. Different, highly specialized forms of radiation therapy (proton beam and episcleral plaque) are currently being compared with surgical enucleation. The radiation therapy methods allow the eye to be saved, but vision after these treatments is markedly impaired.

Staging of ocular melanoma is similar to that used for skin melanomas, but it takes into account diameter in addition to thickness of the primary lesion. Distant metastases are found in about 2% of people at the time of diagnosis and will develop in another 30–40% of people over time. As with cutaneous melanoma, the risk of developing metastases is directly related to the stage at diagnosis. Also as with cutaneous melanoma, patients have been known to develop metastases as long as 40 years after effective treatment of the primary lesion.

Ocular melanoma differs from melanoma arising on the skin, however, in that it almost always spreads to the liver first. In fact, medical students are taught to think of ocular melanoma in any patient with a glass eye and an enlarged liver, and blood tests monitoring the liver are an important part of follow-up visits. Unfortunately, no treatment (and many have been tried) has been shown to be of benefit in the treatment of ocular melanoma that has spread beyond the eye. For this reason, we do not recommended that a person with metastatic ocular melanoma undergo further treatment unless it is part of a research study investigating a new form of therapy that could prove beneficial.

Leptomeningeal Melanoma

Leptomeninges is the medical name for the membranes covering the brain and spinal cord. Melanocytes reside normally in the leptomeninges, so melanoma may develop there, but it is one of the rarest forms of the disease. Only a few cases have ever been reported. When it does occur, it is often in persons with a giant congenital nevus. Patients often come to their doctors complaining of persistent unexplained headaches (that are usually unlike any headache they have ever had before), numbness, weakness in a leg and/or arm, vision changes, drowsiness, or seizures. Melanoma may be provisionally diagnosed from an MRI scan of the brain, which is commonly performed to evaluate such symptoms. It is usually not confirmed, however, until a sample of fluid removed from the spinal cord (a spinal tap) is examined and reveals the presence of melanoma cells. Spread along the spinal cord is common. No effective treatment has been found, although injection of cytokines into the spinal fluid is being investigated.

LESS COMMON FORMS OF CUTANEOUS MELANOMA

Multiple Primary Melanomas

According to several large studies, 1–8% of people who develop a melanoma of the skin will—when examined over many years—develop multiple primaries. (A *primary*, recall, is a new cancer, usually on the skin.) This is mainly because many parts of the body have been exposed to the same UV damage. It may also be due in part to inheritance of cancer-prone genetic traits, such as the absence or mutation of p16, discussed in Chapter 3.

A report from the Yale Melanoma Clinic described a study of 27 patients who had multiple primary lesions. Twenty-two of the patients had a single second primary, while five patients had three primary lesions. We have seen patients with as many as ten primary lesions.

New primaries often do not develop in the same area of the body as the first lesion. One study found that most second primaries (about 70%) developed on a different part of the body than the initial lesion. About 30% of the time, additional primaries are found when the original melanoma is diagnosed; the rest are found later. The additional primaries in 40% of this latter group are found within the first 3 years, and in 20%, they are found between 3 and 7 years later. Importantly, however, 40% of new primaries are not discovered until more than 7 years after the original lesion.

All of this means that all patients with a primary melanoma require a thorough and complete skin examination at the time of original diagnosis and for many years thereafter—probably for life. Fortunately, subsequent primary melanomas are almost always caught at an earlier stage than the original lesion because of the vigilance of the patient and doctor. Studies have shown that although the first melanomas in these patients average between 2 and 3 millimeters in depth, subsequent lesions are usually less than 1 millimeter deep.

People at greatest risk for development of multiple primaries are those with the atypical mole syndrome, those with a family history of melanoma, and older males. Thirty-five percent of patients with the atypical mole syndrome who have developed one primary lesion will develop one or more additional primary melanomas during the following 10 years. This shows just how high the risk in this group is and emphasizes again the need for continued high-level follow-up care. Currently, there is not enough data to quantify the risk of additional melanomas for melanoma patients with p16 mutations, but the incidence of multiple primaries in this group is clearly higher than in melanoma patients without this mutation. Why older males are at higher risk for multiple primaries has not been determined.

It has also been shown that 15% of patients who develop more than one primary lesion, even if they don't have a family history of melanoma, will have an inherited mutation of the p16 gene. This has raised the questions of whether all patients with multiple primary melanomas should be tested for p16 gene mutations and whether other family members should be examined for unrecognized melanomas. Until further data are available, we can give no firm recommendations on these questions, but if you have multiple primaries, you might want to discuss the issue with your physician.

Acral Lentiginous Melanoma

Most skin contains hair, although it may be sparse, fine, and not easily seen. The only exceptions are the palms of the hands, the soles of the feet, and the skin under the fingernails and toenails. The dark pinkish-red linings of the mouth, anus, rectum, vagina, and insides of the eyelids also do not contain hair. Melanoma arising in these areas is called **acral lentiginous melanoma.** *Acral* means "non-hair-bearing." *Lentiginous* is a word describing the distinctive fashion in which the cancer cells in this type of melanoma tend to line up under the microscope.

The cause of acral lentiginous melanoma is not known. It is probably not related to sun exposure because these areas receive little if any sun. Two to eight percent of Caucasian melanoma cases are acral lentiginous melanoma, and there is a substantially higher proportion of cases among blacks, Asians, and Hispanics. This does not mean that the number of cases in these latter groups is high; it only means that they are very unlikely to develop other types of cutaneous melanoma.

MELANOMA OF THE PALMS AND SOLES

The skin on the palms and soles is very thick, and melanoma beginning in these sites is often not noticed at first. In addition, we seldom look at the soles of our feet—unlike, say, the skin on our forearms and face, which we view every day. Eventually, though, melanoma on the soles or palms will become readily visible as a brown or black spot that may even break through the skin and bleed. Often by the time a diagnosis is made, the melanoma has penetrated deeply under the skin, increasing the likelihood for spread to other sites in the body. For this reason, melanoma on the palms and especially the soles has a poor prognosis overall. If it is caught and treated early, however, the prognosis is similar to other skin melanomas and is staged and treated in the same way.

The sole of the foot is the most common site for acral lentiginous melanoma. Patients frequently give a history of trauma to the area, such as stepping on a nail or a thorn or finding an irritant in their shoe, before the melanoma arose. We don't know whether such trauma is in any way related to the development of the melanoma or whether it simply brings attention to the area, leading to the discovery of the lesion.

MELANOMA UNDER THE FINGERNAILS OR TOENAILS
(SUBUNGUAL MELANOMA)

Subungual melanoma is the name given to those uncommon melanomas that arise under the fingernails and toenails. They occur in both Caucasians and non-Caucasians. The diagnosis is often preceded by a long history of what was thought to be a chronic nail infection. If the primary lesion begins where the nail begins its growth, a black streak may appear along the nail. Sometimes there is also pigment found along the border between the beginning of the fingernail and the skin of the finger itself, near the cuticle. Treatment is amputation of the toe or finger, followed by the same close follow-up as recommended for cutaneous primaries.

MELANOMA OF THE MOUTH OR GUMS

Melanoma arising in the lining of the mouth or gums is rare. It occurs most often in Asians, who have more melanocytes and pigmentation in these areas than people of other races. We don't know the cause of this melanoma, but as in most other unusual melanomas, it is probably not sun exposure. Staging and treatment are the same as for skin melanoma, but the prognosis is less favorable for reasons that we do not yet know.

MELANOMA OF THE ANUS, RECTUM, AND VAGINA

Melanoma of the rectum and anus is also rare (only one case per million people is reported each year) and seems to occur randomly. There is no known relationship to environmental factors, lifestyle, or family history. It strikes males and females equally, usually at an older age than skin melanoma. Often patients experience pain and itching and think they have hemorrhoids. These symptoms, however, are really caused by the developing anal melanoma. Certainly hemorrhoids are by far the most common cause of anal pain or itching, but if these symptoms persist despite adequate treatment of hemorrhoids, you should have the region examined by a specialist. Because they are located internally and thus are not readily visible, rectal melanomas have often penetrated deeply by the time they are diagnosed. They therefore usually carry a grave prognosis. Treatment is surgical excision. Elective regional lymph node resection at the time of diagnosis does not improve outcome, and it is not recommended unless the lymph nodes are enlarged.

Melanoma of the penis is extremely rare, but vaginal melanoma occurs more often, in adult females of all ages and racial origins, and has no known relationship to environmental factors, sun exposure, infection, lifestyle, or family background. Melanoma may arise on the outer lips of the vagina (the vulva) or it may arise inside the vagina. Moles may occur on the inside or outside of the vulvar lips, and they may develop into melanoma, just like moles anywhere else on the body. Melanomas inside the vagina, however, may appear without a preexisting nevus. They may be flat or raised and often create a sensation of itching. They may even be multiple. Staging is slightly different than for skin melanoma, but treatment is similar, with early surgical excision being the primary step. The effectiveness of elective surgical lymph node dissection is under debate. Prognosis for these melanomas is, stage for stage, no different than prognosis for skin melanoma, but these melanomas often have penetrated deeply by the time of diagnosis.

For anal, rectal, and vaginal melanomas, recurrence in the local area is often more common than internal metastases. This sounds like a good thing, but unfortunately, local recurrences may be so aggressive that they can cause a lot of problems. Patients often require repeated surgeries, which must sometimes be very extensive. A *pelvic exoneration*—surgical removal of the entire bladder, rectum, and sexual organs—may be necessary.

Amelanotic Melanoma

We described this form of melanoma in Chapter 4. When melanomas are not pigmented they are often missed because neither the patient nor the doctor considers the possibility of melanoma when they observe the lesion. Nonetheless, 3–5% of all melanomas are amelanotic. If you have an uncolored or lightly colored lesion that appears to be a pimple or bite but does not go away within 4 weeks, consult your physician. You should probably have it removed and examined by a pathologist. Amelanotic melanoma is no more dangerous than other melanomas except that there is a greater likelihood that you will not notice it as quickly. Treatment is the same as for other melanomas.

Cutaneous Lesions That May Develop into Melanoma

SPITZ NEVUS

Spitz nevus is the name given to a type of mole which most often arises in children and young adults and which can be confused with melanoma. In fact, another name for *Spitz nevus* is *benign juve-*

nile melanoma, but this is a contradiction of terms, since melanoma is never benign. Spitz nevi are usually small (less than 1 centimeter across), round, and dome-shaped, and they have well-defined borders and may be slightly scaly. They are usually tan, pink, or red, but they may also be brown or black. They occur most often on the face and legs, although they may occur anywhere. They seem to be more common in girls than boys. They usually arise quite rapidly over a few months and tend to persist for life. One-third arise in children under 10; one-third arise between the ages of 10–20; and one-third arise after age 20, but, like all nevi, they rarely arise after age 30. The most important thing about Spitz nevi is that when examined under a microscope, they have features similar to melanoma. It is often a challenge even for experts to distinguish between the two.

True Spitz nevi are completely benign. Only a few cases of melanoma arising in a Spitz nevus have been reported. Because of the difficulty in distinguishing them from melanoma with 100% certainty, however, it is always safest to treat the mole in this case as if it were melanoma by removing it along with a rim of normal tissue around the lesion (wide local excision). (See Franco's story below.)

MALIGNANT BLUE NEVUS

Blue nevi, sometimes called *blue dome nevi,* are just what they sound like: raised, dome-shaped dark blue moles. They are usually found on the head or scalp and are often present from birth. They only rarely develop into melanoma, but when they do, they have peculiar features not seen with most other melanomas. The most important of these is local spread into the surrounding skin after the primary lesion has been removed. This is evidenced by the appearance of multiple small blue lumps or nodules around the scar of the excision site. Further surgery is often followed by reappearance and continued local spread with subsequent development of lymph node and distant metastases that are highly refractory to any known therapy. The recommended treatment for any blue dome nevus that might be malignant is immediate wide local excision.

MELANOMA ARISING IN GIANT CONGENITAL NEVI

We described giant congenital nevi in Chapter 2. The major concern, other than cosmetic, for these nevi is the risk of their developing into melanoma. This occurs in 5–10% of large lesions (those bigger than 20 centimeters in diameter) and in 1% or less of small lesions. Half of the melanomas arising in the large nevi develop in childhood. It is not clear whether this risk is enhanced by excessive sun exposure. All patients with large lesions should be seen by a specialist at regular intervals. When melanoma does occur, it does not arise in the entire lesion. Rather, it occurs in a small area and grows from there. Worrisome areas should be biopsied. If melanoma is found, a wide excision is done around the affected area. Further management is similar to that for melanoma arising in a common acquired nevus.

Unusual Populations for Melanoma

As we have said repeatedly, most melanoma occurs in fair-skinned Caucasian adults. Because *most* is not *all,* everyone should watch for the warning signs of the disease.

Melanoma in Children

Melanoma in childhood is uncommon because most moles do not develop until puberty. There is, in fact, a common misconception in the medical community and among the general public that melanoma does not occur in children at all. Parents' concerns about pigmented lesions on their children are often dismissed by the children's doctors, and observation of the number of moles a child has and their characteristics is not a part of a routine physical.

In recent years, however, as the general incidence of the disease has risen, more and more children have been diagnosed with melanoma. This is probably because more children are being exposed to more sun earlier and are therefore developing nevi at younger ages. Studies of young children have shown that those living in sunny climates develop moles in larger numbers and at younger ages than those living farther from the equator.

Parents and physicians must begin to pay more attention to children's moles, especially since two of the factors that put people most at risk for the development of melanoma (a large number of moles and atypical moles) can be easily identified by the child's teenage years—

a time when UV protection and scrupulous observation of moles would have the greatest impact in preventing melanoma. Children in families with a history of melanoma should be watched especially carefully. Children with a parent or sibling who has had melanoma are at an increased risk of developing the disease. This is probably the result of a complex interaction of factors, including inheritance of skin type, inheritance of genetic mutations, and following similar lifestyles.

Melanoma in children under 5 years old is very uncommon and usually develops in a congenital nevus, particularly in a giant hairy nevus, as we have seen. In older children and teenagers, melanoma usually begins in moles acquired after birth, as it does in adults. Treatment and outcome of these melanomas are also the same as for adults. Melanoma is the most common cancer of the eye in children, but even so, it is very rare.

Franco's Story

The end of Franco's story was related in Chapter 10. Here is how the story began: When Franco was 12, his mother became concerned about a dark mole on his back. She took Franco to his regular doctor to have it examined. The doctor told them it was a Spitz nevus and that, anyway, "Kids don't get melanoma." It was only a year later, when the mole continued to change, that the doctor agreed to remove it. Several pathologists looked at the specimen, but they did not agree. Some said it was melanoma, while others believed it was merely a Spitz nevus. They all agreed, however, that it should be treated as melanoma, and so the skin around the mole was removed.

When Franco began getting lumps under the skin near the site of the original mole, his doctor reassured his parents that the lumps had nothing to do with the mole. When they were eventually removed and biopsied, however, the lumps were found to contain melanoma. The melanoma eventually spread to Franco's lymph nodes and to most of his internal organs as well as his brain. Despite numerous operations, chemotherapy, and radiation treatments, Franco's condition deteriorated. He became so

There has been an increase in the number of cases of melanoma reported in children in recent years. In Australia, there has been a concerted effort to get children out of the sun by requiring use of sun-protective clothing at | *The rising incidence of melanoma in children*

primary schools, by holding outdoor activities in either the early morning or the late afternoon hours (when the sun is less intense), and by mounting aggressive public education campaigns.

Recent statistics from Australia have shown the benefit of these efforts. Although the incidence of melanoma has continued to increase in older adults, whose sun exposure occurred in past years, it is beginning to decrease in people under the age of 30. Education of children about the dangers of sun exposure by parents, physicians, and teachers should be done repeatedly and routinely.

weak he could no longer walk and had trouble breathing. He was only 16 when he died.

Of course, no one knows whether Franco would have survived if the nevus on his back had been removed at the first visit. Fortunately, tragic stories like this are uncommon. We have told the story, however, to underline the fact that it is never too early to check children for moles and to insist that any moles that concern you be removed.

Melanoma in Pregnant Women

It is common for moles to become darker or to grow during pregnancy, probably because of the effects of hormones on melanocytes. Indeed, during puberty (when hormone levels also rise), there is an increase in mole number. These same factors occasionally seem to stimulate an apparently benign mole to develop into melanoma. One to two percent of all melanomas in women are diagnosed during pregnancy. Unless there is evidence of metastases beyond the primary site, requiring further therapy, there is no reason to terminate the pregnancy. This is because wide local excision of the primary lesion can be carried out safely without any effect on the developing fetus. If there are no abnormal findings on physical examination, no abnormal blood tests, and no symptoms to suggest the melanoma may have spread internally, radiological studies should be put on hold until after the baby is delivered, to avoid exposing the fetus to the potentially harmful effects of radiation.

In the rare instance where metastases are present at the time of diagnosis, the decision whether or not to terminate the pregnancy will depend on the stage of the melanoma, the length of time before delivery can be safely accomplished, and the treatment required. Early termination of pregnancy has no apparent effect on the progression of the melanoma. Transmission of melanoma to the fetus has been reported, but it is extremely rare and occurs only when the mother has very widespread metastases.

Studies have shown that the prognosis for women diagnosed with melanoma during pregnancy is no different from that for non-pregnant women of the same age with similar melanomas. In both cases, the prognosis depends on the site and the stage of the melanoma when it is diagnosed.

Women who have developed melanoma while pregnant often ask, "If I get pregnant again, will I develop another melanoma, or worse yet, will it stimulate any melanoma cells that may have escaped into my bloodstream to grow into metastatic tumors?" This is a very good and important question for women who desire subsequent pregnancies. Unfortunately, no studies have been done to answer this question satisfactorily. Because the majority of recurrences of melanoma occur in the first 2–3 years after diagnosis, most specialists recommend that women diagnosed with melanoma, whether during pregnancy or not, wait at least 3 years before becoming pregnant (see also Chapter 7).

Melanoma in Non-Caucasians

Melanoma can occur in all racial and ethnic groups. The incidence is directly related to skin color—the lighter your skin, the higher your likelihood of developing melanoma. For white Americans, more than 1 in 100 persons will develop melanoma in their lifetime. For blacks, fewer than 1 in 10,000 will ever develop melanoma. For other races, the lifetime incidence is somewhere in between. The

Darkening of the skin, particularly around the nipples and on the cheeks, is common during pregnancy. Moles also frequently become darker or larger, or may be noted for the first time during pregnancy. These phenomena are | *Changes in pigmentation during pregnancy*

not in themselves worrisome; they are just normal responses to the many hormonal changes occurring in the body. Patients and physicians alike, however, should be aware that melanoma may also show up during pregnancy, probably as a result of the same hormonal changes. Pregnancy also causes some suppression of the immune system to prevent it from attacking the developing fetus. This, too, may be related to the development of melanoma at this time. Any mole that continues to change or that changes asymmetrically or irregularly during pregnancy should be removed. This can be done safely with local anesthetic without harm to the developing fetus.

incidence of melanoma has not increased in blacks in recent decades as it has in whites. There are early indications, however, that the incidence of melanoma is beginning to rise in Hispanics, although the total numbers remain low.

When melanoma does develop in nonwhites, it is frequently in areas of the body that are the lightest in color. In blacks, melanoma occurs almost exclusively on the palms of the hands and the soles of the feet. In Asians, the gums are a frequent site of melanoma. Melanoma in desert-dwelling Arabs most commonly arises on the face and nose, presumably the result of intense sun exposure of these areas while the rest of the body is fully covered. The body distribution of melanoma in Hispanics is similar to that seen in white populations.

Melanoma in Albino People

Albino persons are people with no pigment in their bodies. Their hair is white, their eyes are pink, their skin is extremely fair, and they have no pigmented nevi. You would think, then, that they could not develop melanoma, but they do, and not uncommonly. This is because the white skin of albinos stems not from an absence of melanocytes, which they have in normal numbers, but rather from the inability of their melanocytes to make melanin pigments. This lack of protective pigmentation makes them more prone to all types of skin cancer. Because the melanomas that develop in albino persons are not pigmented, they are often overlooked until they become large and raised. Any changing skin lesion on the skin of an albino person should be considered suspicious and promptly removed and biopsied.

Melanoma in Immunocompromised People

People whose immune systems have been weakened by disease or treatment with medicines that affect the function of the immune system are said to be **immunocompromised.** Included in this group are people infected with the AIDS virus (HIV), patients who have had an organ transplant, and those with lupus, rheumatoid arthritis, cancer, or other diseases that require treatment with steroids, chemotherapy drugs, or other medications that suppress the immune system. All of these patients have a higher incidence of melanoma and other cancers than people of similar age, sex, and race who do not have these conditions.

When melanoma develops in these patients, it often emerges rather suddenly and appears to grow rapidly. Treatment is similar to that given to patients who are not immunocompromised. In addition, any medications that suppress the immune system should be stopped when this is feasible. Anyone infected with the AIDS virus should be treated with the aggressive multidrug regimens that have proven effective in suppressing the virus and improving the functioning of the immune system.

Data showing that people with suppressed immune systems are at an increased risk for developing melanoma are so new that we do not yet know how their prognosis compares with that of the general population. Unfortunately, it is probably worse, particularly if medications used to suppress the immune system cannot be stopped.

Melanoma in Animals

Most animals have a protective covering of hair over their skin and are less likely to develop melanoma than humans. Melanoma does, however, develop in many domestic and farm animals, including dogs, horses, cattle, swine, mice, and fish. In dogs, melanoma most commonly occurs in the gums and mouth, especially in breeds such as chows that have pigmented gums. Hereford cattle frequently develop ocular melanoma, particularly when raised outdoors at high altitudes. Melanoma of the rectum and anus occurs in horses, most often grays. One breed of pigs called Sinclair swine have moles and thus a predilection for developing melanoma of the skin just like humans. Various types of melanoma have been developed in mice and fish in the laboratory to help find and test methods of treatment that may be of benefit to humans.

Indeed, there is a great deal of research going on in laboratories and clinics throughout the world aimed at improving the prevention, diagnosis, and treatment of melanoma. In the next chapter, we shall describe the major areas that are being explored and what this research may mean for melanoma patients.

13

What's New in Melanoma Research?

Y ou will have noticed that many of the treatments covered in Chapter 10 are still experimental. Experimental treatments are being tested all the time, since research into the cause and treatment of malignant melanoma is progressing at a rapid pace at medical centers throughout the world. The growth of new knowledge is so great that we can cover only the highlights in this chapter. Even these will be somewhat out of date by the time this book is published because new realizations and new treatment options are reported almost every day.

A search of the medical literature shows that 2,056 scientific articles dealing with all aspects of melanoma were published in 1999 alone, and the number of studies continues to grow. Scientists from a wide range of fields are attacking the problem from many different angles. Researchers include physicists, atmospheric scientists, geneticists, molecular and cell biologists, surgeons, and oncologists.

Researchers publish their findings in medical journals, one of which deals exclusively with the problem of melanoma. Among the most prominent of these journals are *Melanoma Research, Nature, Cancer Research,* the *Journal of Investigative Dermatology, Cancer,* the *Journal of the American Medical Association, Lancet,* the *Journal of Clinical Oncology,* and the *New England Journal of Medicine.* In addition, at regular national and international meetings researchers present papers on their work and discussion among scientists allows for an easy exchange of new ideas, data, and research materials.

Several laboratories often collaborate on large clinical research projects, each laboratory researching a different aspect of a single problem. These collaborations are easier now because of the Internet and e-mail. It is unlikely that any one scientist or group will develop a miracle cure for melanoma overnight because major advances come only from the long, hard slogging away in laboratories and clinics of many dedicated scientists and physicians. Like the health-care workers who work with melanoma patients, these scientists and physicians share the frustrations and dreams of all the melanoma sufferers who long for a cure for this terrible disease. In this chapter, we will discuss some of the current areas of study in this battle and how such studies may affect the care of melanoma patients in the future.

We have divided this chapter into two sections, one dealing with laboratory research and the other with clinical research. Although the two kinds of research often overlap, there are important differences. Laboratory research is done in test tubes and other laboratory containers or using experimental animals. Clinical research, on the other hand, is the direct study of and investigative treatment of patients with the disease. Clinical research includes studies of who gets the disease and why, devising and testing new surgical and diagnostic techniques, and of course the testing of new treatments.

You may hear laboratory studies described as *in vitro* (literally, "in glass") and clinical studies described as *in vivo* ("in that which is alive"). This is an important distinction because, while in vitro studies are frequently the necessary prelude to in vivo studies, many treatments that work in the test tube do not perform as well in animal studies or in the human body.

Most of the laboratory research, and much of the clinical research, takes place in large medical centers and research institutions. New experimental therapies, however, are often available through physicians in communities throughout the world who participate in large cooperative group studies. If you have melanoma, you may be asked to participate in one of the many studies under way, thus becoming part of the research effort yourself. (We'll discuss this further below.)

LABORATORY RESEARCH IN MELANOMA

The Genes and Genetics of Melanoma

There has been an explosion in knowledge about the genetics of human disease during the past 25 years. Basic research into the structure of DNA and rapid advances in computer technology have transformed what were once tedious, time-consuming, and often impossible investigations into procedures that are performed with ease in laboratories across the world. If you have melanoma or are close to someone who has, you may wish that scientists would spend less time studying genetics and more time testing possible cures. With cells as complex and variable as melanoma cells, however, it is only through understanding exactly how and why the disease develops and spreads that we are likely to find treatments that do more than delay its devastating activity.

You will remember from Chapter 1 that genes are stretches of precise DNA sequences that instruct the body to produce a certain protein. All together, our genes are responsible for making us human beings but at the same time different from any other human being that ever did or ever will exist. Most cancers are the result of errors or mutations in one or more of these genes. At present, we know the function of only a fraction of our 100,000 genes.

Among the genes whose function we have partially uncovered are several that are involved in the development and progression of cancer, including melanoma. These cancer-related genes have so far been grouped into two large categories, **oncogenes** and **tumor suppressor genes.** To understand their actions and the difference between them, recall that the precise quantity of all cells in the body is carefully regulated. You do not want too many or too few of any cell type. **Proto-oncogenes** and tumor suppressor genes are *normal* genes that provide blueprints for the proteins that control cell proliferation and make certain that the precise cell number of each cell type is maintained at all times.

The proteins made by proto-oncogenes instruct the cell to divide. When the proper cell division is complete, the protein disintegrates. An oncogene is a proto-oncogene gone bad. In other words, the precise sequence of DNA in the proto-oncogene has been altered, or mutated, say from ultraviolet light, and this damage interferes with the normal functioning of the gene. This may result in a protein that is more active or more long-lasting, so that the cells it stimulates divide more rapidly than they should. It is a bit like having the gas pedal on your car stuck to the floor at all times—likely to lead to a crash or, in the case of cells, a tumor.

Tumor suppressor genes were described briefly in Chapter 3. They work in combination with proto-oncogenes. They are more like the brakes on your car. The proteins they encode *inhibit* cell division. When these genes are damaged or destroyed, cell proliferation can also speed up, like your car on a hill with no brakes. Although damage to both of these types of genes has been implicated in the development and progression of melanoma, we will concentrate on tumor suppressor genes, because they seem to play a bigger role.

CURRENT RESEARCH ON THE P16 GENE

In Chapter 3, we described how researchers discovered the high correlation between missing or damaged p16 genes and melanoma. Now that scientists have isolated this problem, they have been working on ways to compensate for the missing or damaged p16 gene. In the laboratory, it has been shown that reintroduction of a normal p16 gene into cells lacking it can restore some growth control. This process of putting good copies of genes into cells that have bad copies is called **gene therapy.**

The obvious question, then, is why not use gene therapy with p16 to prevent or cure melanoma in people who lack this gene? Unfortunately, right now that is a monumental task. First of all, it is much easier to insert a gene artificially into a cell when the cell is sitting in a dish on a laboratory bench than when the cell is in the center of a tumor, say in the lung, bone, or brain. Secondly, the gene would have to be inserted into all, or nearly all, of the billions of melanocytes in the normal human being, because it only takes a single malignant melanocyte to generate a massive tumor. As if that weren't enough, the gene must get into an exact place in the long stretches of DNA in each and every cell, and it must be regulated in some way so that it doesn't work too fast or too slow.

These are just a few of the obstacles that must be overcome before gene therapy will work. For the moment, unfortunately, gene therapy is just not possible in melanoma. Current research is aimed mainly at determining precisely how p16 works. The hope is that once we know this, we can devise methods to substitute for its loss, perhaps with specially designed drugs or cytokines. This is an area of intense study around the world and is likely to result in important breakthroughs in the future.

A form of gene therapy is currently being tested in melanoma patients, but only with genes that act by enhancing immune attack against melanoma cells. We will discuss this in the clinical research section below.

OTHER GENES IN MELANOMA

It is clear that p16 is only one of many genes whose mutation or loss is responsible for the development of melanoma. We know this because 85% of families with hereditary melanoma seem to have totally normal p16 genes. Although p16 is important because it was the first to be found and studied in detail, an intense search is under way for other genes that we know must be involved. Initial studies have suggested that genes residing on chromosomes 1 and 8 may be important, but these genes have yet to be identified. The pace of the search is picking up, however, with the work of the Human Genome Project, a massive project ongoing at several major research centers that is dedicated to identifying the structure and sequence of the entire human genome—all of the human genes. As the Human Genome Project continues, it is likely that these and other melanoma-related genes will be identified in the next few years.

Meanwhile, other investigators are concentrating on the oncogenes, particularly one called *ras*. Ras is often mutated and "turned on" in melanoma cells, and often in the same cells that have loss of p16 function. The effect of these two mutations in conjunction is like losing the brakes in your car with the gas pedal pushed to the floor. For the moment, no one knows how to turn ras off effectively, but there are suggestions that it may be possible.

Cytokine Regulation of Melanocytes and Melanoma Cells

Cytokines are the chemicals released by one cell to signal or regulate neighboring cells. We have already described two cytokines, alpha interferon and interleukin-2, that regulate the cells of the immune system (Chapters 9 and 10). Similar cytokines regulate normal melanocytes. For example, when you expose your skin to the sun, particularly intense sun, the cells in the outer layer of the skin make and send protein messages back to the melanocytes saying, "Hey, we're getting burned out here! Send us some more melanin." Other cytokines make certain that melanocytes do not divide unless there is a good reason to.

Scientists have identified a number of cytokines that contribute to the well-being and proper functioning of melanocytes. Among those identified so far are *stem cell factor* (SCF), the *endothelins 1 and 3, melanocyte-stimulating hormone* (MSH), and *fibroblast growth factor* (FGF). Melanocytes have specific receptors on their surfaces to which these cytokines must attach in order to transmit their messages. If the receptors are missing or damaged, no message can get through. When melanoma develops, these receptors begin to disappear from the cell surface. Fewer and fewer cytokine messages get through, and another set of normal controls is lost. Now your car has no brakes, the gas pedal is at full throttle, and no one can hear your calls for help—a disastrous combination.

Much current research is aimed at identifying additional melanocyte-related cytokines and determining exactly how they work, what leads to their production, and why their receptors are lost with the development of melanoma. Researchers have identified the genes for the cytokines listed above and their receptors and have generated them in the laboratory. This will open the way to a better understanding of how normal melanocytes are regulated and how we can use this knowledge to control melanoma cells in patients who have the disease.

The Immune System and Melanoma

During the past 25 years, no area of melanoma research has received more attention than the immune system. The occasional spontaneous disappearance of melanoma without treatment, a few successes with immunotherapy, and the rapid advances that have been made in our general understanding of the immune system have fueled hopes that work on the immune system will be the source of a cure. The focus of this research is to determine why the immune system fails to destroy melanoma tumor cells and then to use this knowledge to develop effective specific melanoma immunotherapy. It is amply clear from many previous studies that simply "boosting" the immune system nonspecifically is unlikely to be useful (see Chapter 9).

The immune system may be unable to cope with melanoma

partly because of damage to a unique set of immune cells that reside in the skin, called *dendritic cells*. Current thinking is that the loss, damage, or suppression of these cells may allow melanoma to develop. Laboratory tests using animal models have shown that intense UV light markedly suppresses these dendritic immune cells at the same time that it damages the DNA of the nearby melanocytes. Scientists are now studying ways to rescue or restore the skin's dendritic and other immune cells.

We have already mentioned that people whose immune systems have been damaged or suppressed by the AIDS virus or by drugs to prevent rejection of transplanted organs or to treat certain diseases have an increased risk of developing melanoma. In the vast majority of melanoma patients, however, no abnormalities in the functioning of the immune system can be demonstrated. The problem is not that the immune system is not functioning; the problem is that it isn't functioning at a specific level—the level at which it might recognize the melanoma cells as foreign, and attack and destroy them. How can we overcome this problem? The answer is being sought through specific immunotherapy.

Research in this area is aimed at finding antigens made by melanoma cells that are not made (or are made only in small amounts) by normal cells and using these proteins to make melanoma vaccines (see Chapter 9). The idea is to identify these "melanoma-specific antigens," prepare them in a form that will look foreign and attractive to the immune system, inject them in the skin, and let the onslaught begin. The hope is that once the immune cells have been primed by exposure to these antigens, they will proliferate and travel around the body, like a swarm of bees seeking and killing any cells that display the antigens. A large number of these melanoma-specific antigens have been found and reproduced in the laboratory. They are now being tested for their effectiveness in humans.

A somewhat similar approach is to generate antibodies that recognize these antigens in the laboratory and inject the antibodies instead of the antigens. Individual antibodies recognizing the antigen of your choice can be produced in large quantities in the laboratory; antibodies made in this way are called **monoclonal antibodies.** Large numbers of these antibodies are injected into a vein and circulate in the bloodstream until they come across melanoma cells with the target antigen on their surface. The antibodies then attach to the antigens. This alerts other immune cells to move in and do the killing. A variation on this technique is to attach a toxic substance or a radioisotope to the antibody—a sort of "poison pill"—so that when the antibody attaches to its target antigen, the poison is delivered directly to the melanoma cell.

Unfortunately, each of these approaches faces major theoretical and technical difficulties: not all melanoma cells produce the same antigens, many of the antigens they do produce are also made by normal cells, the immune system is reluctant to go after its own family of cells, and its response is often weak and ineffective. To overcome these problems, researchers are experimenting with combining immune cytokines with the vaccines and altering their protein structure to make them more active.

Studies in Melanoma Metastases

We know that melanoma cells circulate throughout the bloodstream in many patients. What is puzzling is that only a small fraction of these cells are eventually able to settle down and grow into a new tumor in some other place in the body. Even more puzzling is the fact that they like to grow, at least initially, only in certain organs, even though they must pass through all of them. Melanoma cells, for example, rarely ever stop to grow in the kidney, which has one of the highest rates of blood flow in the body. They proliferate instead in the liver, brain, and lungs. The explanation for this is undoubtedly complex, and it is of great current interest.

If we could prevent the attachment and growth of melanoma cells before they got a foothold, we could conceivably prevent metastases from ever developing. As we mentioned in Chapter 9, before a melanoma cell can metastasize in an organ, it must first adhere to that organ and set up blood and cytokine supplies. Researchers are studying each of these steps and looking for ways to prevent them. They have been able to describe the *adhesion molecules* made by melanoma cells, which allow them to stick to the walls of blood vessels, and are investigating ways to rid the cells of these molecules. They have isolated *angiogenesis factors* made by melanoma cells, which allow the formation of new blood vessels. Clinical trials of compounds that inhibit these factors are now under way. Finally, scientists have identified many of the cytokines needed to keep melanoma cells healthy, and they are now exploring ways of suppressing their production. Most of these areas of study remain at the laboratory stage, but a few tentative approaches at treatment in humans are under way.

CLINICAL RESEARCH IN MELANOMA

Better and Easier Diagnosis

Everyone agrees that if we could figure out which atypical moles were going to turn into melanoma, we could prevent more cases. Likewise, if we knew whether or not lymph nodes contained melanoma without invasive surgery, we could give patients better treatment. Techniques to do these things are on the drawing board. Some are even in your doctor's office.

EPILUMINESCENCE

A major problem in evaluating pigmented skin lesions, particularly in people with many moles, is determining which ones to remove and when. Currently, this is done by removing the lesions that concern the doctor or the patient or by taking a baseline set of whole body photographs and removing only the moles that are new or appear to have changed. Although few deep melanomas are missed by these techniques, they often lead to the removal of many benign moles, leaving a frustrated dermatologist, an unhappy patient with many scars, and a nervous insurance company. This is because, even with years of experience, it is not always possible for a doctor to tell with certainty from a mole's appearance on the skin whether it is benign, premalignant, or even frankly malignant.

New techniques are becoming available that may make it easier to distinguish between benign and suspicious nevi, and others are being studied. The best-known new technique is **epiluminescence microscopy.** This technique combines a very bright light and magnification to penetrate the deeper layers of skin and create a magnified image of a mole that may then be projected on a computer screen. These images can then be stored in the computer where they will be available for comparison with new images of the same mole to see whether it has changed. Although epiluminescence microscopy is now available in many major skin centers and doctors' offices, many specialists find it too cumbersome and time-consuming for routine use. For now, it is probably best reserved for patients with the atypical mole syndrome who have a history of developing severely atypical or even malignant moles that show only subtle changes on the skin's surface.

BLOOD TESTS FOR MELANOMA

Most of the blood tests that are available for patients with a history of melanoma do not directly detect the presence of melanoma in the body. Rather, they check on the function of various organs, including the liver, kidneys, and bone marrow. If any of the findings are abnormal, there are a multitude of possible causes, only one of which is the presence of melanoma in the affected organ. Because the list of possibilities is long, additional tests, such as scans or biopsies, are almost always required to determine whether or not melanoma is the culprit. Things would be much simpler if there were a more specific blood test for melanoma. Several such tests are now being studied.

Melanoma cells are difficult to detect in the bloodstream, even in patients with melanoma that has spread throughout the body and even when the blood is studied carefully under a microscope. This is because when melanoma cells are present in the blood, they are far outnumbered by the blood cells themselves. Melanoma cells do, however, have unique biochemical characteristics that can be detected by special laboratory techniques. One of these characteristics is the production of an enzyme called **tyrosinase.** The only job tyrosinase has in the body is to help melanocytes produce their melanin pigments. Therefore, tyrosinase is present only in melanocytes and not in any other cells in the body.

Because melanocytes are not found in the bloodstream unless they have become melanoma, testing the blood for the presence of tyrosinase should determine whether or not a patient has melanoma in his or her bloodstream. And indeed, a highly sensitive technique called *PCR* (polymerase chain reaction) has detected the tyrosinase gene in the blood of some melanoma patients, even when X rays and CT scans have failed to show any evidence of metastasis. Studies are now being conducted to determine how reliable the tyrosinase test is and exactly what a positive or negative result means for the patient. For example, researchers are trying to find out if patients with a positive tyrosinase test are more likely to have a recurrence of their melanoma and whether or not they would benefit from systemic treatment as soon as a positive test result is known. Completion of these studies will take many years. For now, the tyrosinase test is still only a research tool.

A similar test is the *S-100 protein test*. S-100, like tyrosinase, is made only by melanocytes and most melanoma cells. In this case, the protein may be detected by using antibodies that will attach to the S-100 protein if it is present. The antibodies are treated with special dyes so those that have attached to melanocytes or melanoma cells can be seen with a scan. Initial test results suggest that this technique may be useful in monitoring the response to treatment in advanced melanoma (the S-100 protein level decreases if there is a good response to the therapy), but its usefulness in monitoring patients for the development of metastases has yet to be shown.

Lymphoscintigraphy and Sentinel Lymph Node Biopsy

Lymphoscintigraphy and sentinel lymph node biopsy are new means of determining more precisely which lymph node area drains the site of a primary melanoma and whether or not those lymph nodes have been invaded by the melanoma. This information is very useful for determining which patients should have their lymph nodes removed at the time of diagnosis and which lymph nodes should be removed. These techniques are now widely used and accepted. They are described in detail in Chapter 9.

New Methods of Treatment: Immunotherapy

We have already said a great deal about immunotherapy in this book. Everyone—patients, doctors, and even the press—wants to believe it will work. It all sounds so logical and appealing. The reality is that currently available immunotherapy used alone is unlikely to benefit the vast majority of patients with advanced melanoma, and to date, it is of only limited benefit in early stages. The disease is too complex and varies too much from patient to patient. Immunotherapy will most likely find its place as part of multifaceted treatment regimens for early, limited metastatic melanoma and advanced melanoma. These regimens will also involve chemotherapy, surgery, radiation, cytokines, and gene therapy. And this is already happening. We will discuss some of these regimens as well as studies of the newer forms of immunotherapy currently being tested as single agents.

TUMOR VACCINES

Most of the current clinical studies using vaccines are focused on their use as adjuvant therapy (see Chapter 9). That is, these vaccines are aimed at preventing recurrence of melanoma after all known sites of disease have been surgically removed. Test subjects are mainly patients with stage II and stage III melanoma. The vaccines are prepared using antigens derived from melanoma cells. Some use several antigens in the same preparation (so-called *polyvalent vaccines*), while others use single antigens (*monovalent vaccines*). Almost all are given as skin injections in solutions that also contain agents to stimulate the immune system. They are usually given on a weekly basis, or sometimes more often, for 6 months to 2 years. Very few side effects have been reported.

Results of a large randomized trial of one such vaccine (called *vaccinia viral oncolysate/melanoma oncolysate*) have already been reported. They showed that stage III melanoma patients treated with the vaccine had a very slight, but not statistically significant, survival advantage compared to those receiving a placebo. The first results of another large study being done in the United States by a large cooperative group involving many different medical centers should be available soon. If this and other studies show that the vaccines are beneficial, studies involving patients with earlier stages of melanoma will probably be designed.

TUMOR IMMUNIZATION USING PEPTIDE ANTIGENS

Melanoma peptides are purified protein antigens derived from melanocytes or melanoma cells. These peptides are simply small pieces of the whole antigen—the part(s) recognized by the immune system. They are currently being tested as vaccines in patients with advanced melanoma. If the treatments are well tolerated and seem to be effective, they will probably then be tested as adjuvant therapy. There are many different types of peptide vaccines under study. Some

are being given alone (monovalent) and some are given in combinations (polyvalent), often with a cytokine such as *GM-CSF* (see below).
Among those under study are *gp100, Melan-A/Mart-1, Mage 1 and
3,* and tyrosinase. The hope is that these peptides will serve as tar-
gets and stimulate a specific set of immune cells called *cytotoxic T-
lymphocytes* (CTLs), whose job it is to identify, attack, and kill "foreign cells" that may be dangerous to the body.

    If CTLs can be activated against peptides, they should also be ac-
tivated against melanoma cells that carry the antigen (from which the
peptide was derived) on their surface. To activate the CTLs, the peptides first have to be picked up by other cells of the immune system
and "presented" to the CTLs in special grooves called the *HLA* (or human leukocyte antigen complex). Only 70% of people have the right
HLA type (A1 and A2) to display, or present, some of these peptides.
The other 30% are not entered into the trials using these vaccines. Initial studies have shown that the CTL immune cells are indeed acti-
vated in some (but not all) patients with melanoma following peptide
vaccinations, but correlation between their activation and partial or
total remission of tumors is not yet clear. These studies are under way
at numerous centers around the world.

MONOCLONAL ANTIBODIES

We described monoclonal antibodies in the laboratory section of
this chapter. A large number of monoclonal antibody studies have already been done or are currently under way. The antibodies are being
tested both for detecting the spread of melanoma and for treating it.
In either case, the goal is to find and make an antibody that will react
only with melanoma cells. Early studies were done using antibodies
produced by mouse cells. Not surprisingly, the human immune system rejected the mouse-made antibodies after a few injections because
it recognized them as "foreign." More recently, "humanized" antibodies have become available for clinical trials.

    For detecting melanoma that has spread, antibodies designed to
attach only to antigens found on melanoma cells are tagged or labeled
with a radioisotope so that they can be tracked in the body by a scanning device. The labeled antibodies are then injected into a vein and
the body is scanned using a machine similar to a CT scanner. This provides a whole-body image with bright spots where the antibodies have

attached to melanoma antigens. To date, the results of this technique have been mixed. It is able to identify large melanoma deposits, but we do not yet know if we can use it to detect smaller groups of cells than we can with conventional techniques such as CT, MRI, and PET scans.

In the treatment studies, the antibodies are labeled with a more powerful radioisotope or a toxic substance to kill the melanoma cell on contact. This is the "poison-pill" approach mentioned earlier in this chapter, in the section describing laboratory research on the immune system. Before starting such treatment, it is necessary to obtain a biopsy specimen of the patient's melanoma cells to be certain that they carry the antigen the antibody is targeting. Although we know that patients may have several kinds of melanoma cells in their bodies, it is necessary only that some of them carry this antigen. The hope is that the initial killing of some cells will set off a big immune reaction that will encompass all of the cancer cells, even the ones that don't carry the target antigen. Trials of this form of treatment are also being conducted at numerous centers, but no reliable data have yet been reported.

GENE THERAPY

The ideal treatment for any disease is to find the genes that are abnormal, defective, or missing, and then fix or replace them. This is called *specific* gene therapy. Human trials of specific gene therapy are under way in a wide variety of human diseases, but most of them are for diseases like cystic fibrosis, in which only a single, well-studied gene is defective. The problem in melanoma is much more complex. Although only one or a few genes may be defective when melanoma begins, by the time it can be diagnosed, many genes have usually gone haywire. Replacing or correcting them all may not be necessary, but those that do need to be replaced would have to be replaced in every melanoma cell. At the moment, this is beyond our technical capabilities. Gene therapy studies in the laboratory, however, have shown that insertion of the p16 gene into melanoma cells that are missing it or contain a damaged copy results in slowed growth and a more normal appearance.

Current gene therapy in people is instead aimed at making melanoma cells even more abnormal by inserting genes that will cause an immune response—*nonspecific* gene therapy. This is done by injecting cytokine genes, particularly two called GM-CSF and M-CSF, into melanoma tumors. These genes are packaged in a way that allows them to enter the melanoma cells. Once the genes enter the melanoma cells, they "instruct" the cell to make the cytokine they encode for and then to release it into the bloodstream. The released cytokine, in turn, sends a message to the immune system to attack and kill the "releasing" melanoma cells.

There are many problems with this technique. First, it is feasible to inject the genes only into tumors that can be reached easily with a needle—usually tumors under the skin or those that can be felt in lymph nodes. Then, not all of the melanoma cells take in the genes. Finally, even in those that do, production of the cytokine "runs down" after a few days or weeks. Researchers hope, however, that if they can stimulate an initial immune response using this method, the patient's immune system will attack even nonsecreting cells and will continue to do so after secretion of the cytokines diminishes.

Other nonspecific gene therapy approaches are being tested in the laboratory, and more are on the horizon.

COMBINING CHEMOTHERAPY AND CYTOKINES

The aim of the new treatment regimens that combine chemotherapy and cytokines is to kill as many melanoma cells as possible with chemotherapy drugs followed by, or combined with, injection of cytokines that stimulate the immune system to come in and "mop up" what is left. Studies of these combinations are being done both in advanced melanoma and as adjuvant therapy in patients at high risk for recurrence. Initial reports are enthusiastic.

In the most intense adjuvant treatment program, patients with stage III melanoma (enlarged lymph nodes) are first given a mixture of chemotherapy drugs combined with the cytokines IL-2 and interferon for 6 weeks. The enlarged lymph nodes are then removed, followed by another 6–8 weeks of the same treatment. Examination of the lymph nodes at the time of surgery has shown disappearance of or reduction in the number of melanoma cells in more than 50% of patients treated in this way. These studies are only in the early stages, however, and long-term benefit has not yet been demonstrated.

Many different combinations of chemotherapy drugs and cytokines are also being tested in patients with more advanced melanoma. Almost all include the chemotherapy drug DTIC and the cytokine alpha interferon. The more intense regimens also include other chemotherapy drugs such as cisplatinum, BCNU, vinblastine, and vindesine, often with IL-2 and tamoxifen. The reported response rates to such treatments is quite high (50–60% partial or complete remission), except in patients with brain metastases, where the treatments have little or no effect. Unfortunately, however, there are also many side effects, and these regimens are tolerated only by patients who are reasonably fit. Because of this, the regimens must be administered by experienced physicians in a hospital setting.

It is still too early to determine the long-term benefit of these programs, and no one regimen appears to be sufficiently superior to any other to recommend it as the best available treatment. A major concern is that patients given this therapy may still be prone to recurrence of their melanoma in the brain, where the treatments have little benefit. This problem is currently being tackled by adding drugs such as temazolamide and fotemustine that do penetrate into the brain, but data from these studies are not yet available.

FINDING OUT MORE

How Do I Become Part of a Research Study?

Many melanoma patients feel they would like to become part of one of the controlled trials that are testing new treatment options. Joining such a study is a long-term commitment, and you must be aware that there is a good chance you will be assigned to the control group. You will probably know whether or not you have actually received the new treatment, but you will not have a choice as to whether you are in the control group or the experimental treatment group.

To find out more, you should ask your doctor whether she or he knows of any studies you may qualify for. You can also call your local or national cancer society (the American Cancer Society in the United States, the Anti-Cancer Councils in Australia, and similar groups in other countries). The National Institutes of Health (NIH) in the United States has a hot line and web pages that may also help you (see Guide to Resources at the end of this book).

Where Are the Best Melanoma Centers?

There are excellent melanoma specialists throughout the United States, Canada, Europe, and Australia. The important thing is to find a physician near you with whom you are comfortable. Even major melanoma clinics and research centers located far away from where you live can be a source of the latest research results for you and your doctor. You may want to travel to one of these centers for a consultation about diagnosis or treatment, or ask your doctor to call for a consultation.

Where Can I Learn More about Melanoma?

We listed some of the major medical journals at the beginning of this chapter. They are available at most major medical center libraries. One of the best sources of information is your local branch of the cancer society, which will have a number of pamphlets and brochures dealing with melanoma and other cancers and can provide you with information about specialized clinics, support groups, and other resources in your area.

There are also many valuable sites on the Internet that provide information about melanoma, support groups, personal experiences, chat lines, and treatment. See the Guide to Resources at the end of this book for more information about reliable organizations and web sites.

Guide to Resources
for People with Cancer

SUPPORT AND ADVOCACY ORGANIZATIONS

United States

American Academy of Dermatology
    930 N. Meacham Road
    Schaumburg, IL 60173
    888-462-DERM/847-330-0230
    http://www.aad.org
    See also the academy's Web site providing melanoma information,
        http://www.derm-infonet.com/melanomanet

American Cancer Society
    National Headquarters
    1599 Clifton Road NE
    Atlanta, GA 30329-4251
    800-227-2345
    http://www.cancer.org

American Society for Dermatologic Surgery
    Toll-free hotline: 1-800-441-2737 during weekday business hours
        (Central Standard Time)
    http://www.asds-net.org/scfactsheet.html

Burger King Cancer Caring Center
    412-622-1212

Cancer Care, Inc.
    1180 Avenue of the Americas
    New York, NY 10036

    800-813-HOPE
    212-221-3300
    212-302-2400 (social services)

Cancer Conquerors Foundation
    800-238-6479

Cancervive
    310-203-9232

Make Today Count, Mid-America Cancer Center
    800-432-2273

National Cancer Institute (NCI)
    Cancer Information Services
    Public Inquiries, Office of Cancer Communication
    31 Center Drive
    Bethesda, MD 20892-2580
    800-4-CANCER (1-800-422-6237)
    TTY: 800-332-8615
    301-402-5874
    FAX no.: CANCERFAX®
    http://cancernet.nci.nih.gov
    Note: The National Cancer Institute is part of the National Institutes
      of Health

The Melanoma Research Foundation
    P.O. Box 747
    San Leandro, CA 94577
    Telephone/FAX 1-800-MRF-1290
    http://www.melanoma.org
    E-mail: mrf@melanoma.org

National Coalition for Cancer Survivorship (NCCS)
    Suite 300, 5th Floor
    1010 Wayne Avenue
    Silver Spring, MD 20910
    888-YES-NCCS (1-888-937-6227)
    301-650-8868

National Hospice Organization
    Suite 307
    1910 North Fort Myer Drive
    Arlington, VA 22209
    800-658-8898

National Institutes of Health. See National Cancer Institute

R.A. Bloch Cancer Foundation, Inc.
("The Cancer Hotline")
816-932-8453

The Skin Cancer Foundation
212-725-5176

The Wellness Community
310-314-2555

Australia

Anti-Cancer Council of Victoria
1 Rathdowne Street
Carlton South, Vic 3053

United Kingdom

Imperial Cancer Research Fund
P.O. Box 123
Lincoln's Inn Fields
London WC2 3PX
0171-242-0200.
http://www.icnet.uk/research/factsheet/skinindx.html

INTERNET RESOURCES

The Web sites listed below are among those we believe to be most helpful. Most of these sites were recommended by the University of Newcastle's *Guide to Internet Resources for Cancer* (http://www.ncl.ac.uk/~nchwww/guides/clinks2s.htm). Although there are many more helpful and legitimate Web sites that you can find on your own by searching, it's important to keep in mind that there are also sites that may contain inaccurate or harmful information.

From time to time Web sites are removed or renamed, so one or more of these sites may no longer be available.

Melanoma

Chrystal's Home Page/Melanoma Story (USA)
http://www.pe.net/~chrystal

Patient-produced site. Includes a description of life with metastatic malignant melanoma and links to various aspects of skin cancer.

Dan's Melanoma Page (USA)
http://www.electriciti.com/~ssei/mel/melanoma.html
Patient-produced site.

Johns Hopkins Oncology Center, Melanoma and Cutaneous Oncology Clinic (Baltimore, Maryland, USA)
http://www.med.jhu.edu/cancerctr/melanoma/main.htm
A National Cancer Institute–designated Comprehensive Cancer Center. Mailing address: The Melanoma and Cutaneous Oncology Clinic, Johns Hopkins Outpatient Center, Dermatology, 6th Floor, 601 N. Caroline Street, Baltimore, MD 21287. Telephone 410-614-1022. FAX 410-955-0123.

MEL-L E-Melanoma Support Group (Association of Online Cancer Resources [ACOR])
http:/www.acor.org/listserv.html?to_do=interact&listname=MEL-L
E-mail discussion list.

Melanoma (American Cancer Society)
http://www3.cancer.org/cancerinfo/res_home.asp?ct=50
On-line booklet including details about diagnosis, staging, and treatment.

Melanoma (CancerNet)
http://imsdd.meb.uni-bonn.de/cancernet/201302.html
Information about the disease, staging, and treatment.

Melanoma Patients' Information Page (by Jeff Patterson, USA)
http://www.mpip.org
Information about melanoma, abstract searches, clinical trials, bulletin board, chat room, patient's network/register, links.

Melanoma Patients' Network (YourDoctor Inc., USA)
http://www.melanoma.net/index.cfm
Includes detailed information about melanoma and treatment. Board-certified surgeons, oncologists, or dermatologists can pay to be listed on the site's doctor referral service.

Mike's Page—The Melanoma Resource Center
http://www.tustison.com/interests1.html
Many links to melanoma-related resources. Includes a melanoma FAQ page.

Northern California Melanoma Center (Saint Francis Memorial Hospital, San Francisco, California, USA)

> http://www.melanomacenter.com
> Includes details about NCMC and services, news and events, and information about melanoma. Mailing address: Northern California Melanoma Center, Saint Francis Memorial Hospital, Fifth Floor, 900 Hyde Street, San Francisco, CA 94109. Telephone 415-353-6535.

Sunscreens May Not Protect Against Melanoma (Medical Sciences Bulletin, Pharminfo)

> http://pharminfo.com/pubs/msb/sunscrn.html

Understanding Malignant Melanoma (CancerBACUP, UK)

> http://www.cancerbacup.org.uk/info/melanoma.htm
> An on-line booklet. Mailing address: 3 Bath Place, Rivington Street, London EC2A 3JR, UK. Telephone 44-0171-696-9003. FAX 44-0-171-696-9002.

What You Need to Know About Melanoma (National Cancer Institute, USA)

> http://rex.nci.nih.gov/WTNK_PUBS/melanoma/index.htm
> Information about the disease, diagnosis, staging, and treatment options.

Skin Cancer

A Brief Introduction to Skin Cancer

> http://www.maui.net/~southsky/introto.html
> Detailed discussion of ultraviolet light and its effects, UV forecasts, and information about various kinds of skin cancer.

Identifying Skin Cancers (Arizona Cancer Center, Tucson)

> http://www.azcc.arizona.edu/www/text_files/education/skin_cancers.html
> Arizona Cancer Center's COPELINE: 800-622-COPE or in Arizona 520-626-7935. E-mail: copeline@azcc.arizona.edu

Screening for Skin Cancer (CancerNet)

> http://imsdd.meb.uni-bonn.de/cancernet/504724.html
> Patient's information.

Skin Cancer (OncoLink, University of Pennsylvania Cancer Center)

> http://oncolink.upenn.edu/disease/skin1
> General information and numerous links.

Skin Cancer: Overview (MedicineNet)

    http://www.medicinenet.com

    Good information about skin cancer, under the "Diseases and Condi-
tions" tab, with links.

Skin Cancer: The Facts (United Kingdom)

    http://www.jas.tj/skincancer

    Information about various types of skin cancer, treatment, skin protec-
tion, links, and an on-line chat room.

Skin Cancer Guide: Medical Information You Really Want to Know (Afraid-
Toask.com)

    http://www.afraidtoask.com/skinCA

    Information about the various types of skin cancer. Includes graphic
pictures together with information about prevention and early
detection.

Skin Cancer (Memorial Sloan-Kettering Cancer Center)

    http://www.mskcc.org/document/WICSKIN.htm

Skin Cancer Zone

    http://www.skin-cancer.com

    Sections for consumers (open access) and health professionals (requires
password). Graphics-intensive.

Support-Group.com

    http://www.support-group.com

    Addresses for support groups for people with diseases and disorders.
For skin cancer, the site is http://www.support-group.com/cgi-bin/
sg/get_links?skin_cancer. Includes links.

United States National Library of Medicine

    http://www.nlm.nih.gov

    Provides access to Medline, a comprehensive medical database with
more than 8 million references in 3,800 journals.

What Is Skin Cancer? (CanCom, Women's Cancer Information Project)

    http://www.eurohealth.ie/cancom/skin02.htm

What You Need to Know about Moles and Dysplastic Nevi (National Cancer Institute, USA)

    http://rex.nci.nih.gov/WTNK_PUBS/moles/index.htm

    Information about moles, the symptoms of melanoma, how to check
moles, and how to protect your skin.

What You Need to Know about Skin Cancer (National Cancer Institute, USA)

    http://rex.nci.nih.gov/WTNK_PUBS/skin/index.htm

    Information about the disease, diagnosis, staging, and treatment options.

Glossary

ABCD criteria—An abbreviation for remembering four key warning signs or characteristics of moles that may signal the development of dysplasia or melanoma. The criteria are **a**symmetry, irregular **b**orders, **c**olor variegation, and large **d**iameter.

Acquired mutation—Damage to a gene that occurs sometime after birth so that not every cell in the body carries the mutation. Acquired mutations may be caused by a carcinogen, or they may occur spontaneously during the process of cell division.

Acquired—Often used in the medical field to describe a lesion, illness, or condition occurring after birth.

Acquired nevi—Moles that arise after birth. Sometimes called common acquired nevi, because they are so common.

Acral—Pertaining to areas of the skin and body covering that do not have hair. Examples are the palms of the hands, the soles of the feet, and the lining of the mouth. Melanoma arising in these areas is called *acral lentiginous melanoma*. This subtype of melanoma occurs most often in non-Caucasian populations, but it may also occur in Caucasians.

Adjuvant therapy—Literally, "helping" or "enhancing" therapy. This treatment is given to cancer patients who no longer have evidence of cancer detectable by blood tests or scanning techniques but who are at high risk for having a cancer recurrence. The treatment is given to try to prevent such a recurrence by killing any microscopic deposits of cancer cells that may be present.

Alpha interferon—A protein made naturally by the body's immune system. When given by injection in doses higher than the body makes naturally, it may be beneficial in treating some melanoma patients.

Amelanotic melanoma—A melanoma that is not colored or pigmented because it does not produce melanin.

Antibodies—Highly specific molecules made naturally by the body's immune system that bind to foreign antigens. Each antibody binds to one and only one specific antigen. When an antibody-antigen interaction occurs, other cells of the immune system are called in to attack and kill any cells harboring the foreign antigen, since they are usually dangerous to the body. Antibodies may also be generated artificially in the laboratory to target any specific antigen. Antibodies made in this way are called *monoclonal antibodies,* and they are often used to help diagnose or treat diseases.

Antigens—Proteins made by all cells that are usually displayed on the cell's outer surface. The cells of the immune system are able to recognize which of these special proteins are part of an individual's body and which are foreign. If the immune cells recognize an antigen as foreign, they mount a complex immune response to destroy all cells carrying that antigen. Antigens found only on melanoma cells are being used to make experimental melanoma vaccines.

Atypical mole syndrome—A syndrome in which affected persons have more than 100 moles, at least 10 of which have precancerous ("atypical") features. People with this syndrome have a significantly increased risk of developing melanoma. Also called *dysplastic nevus syndrome* and *familial atypical mole and melanoma syndrome,* or FAMM.

Atypical mole—A mole that either looks abnormal on the skin and/or has precancerous features when removed and looked at under a microscope. Atypical moles are associated with an increased risk of melanoma, and some will eventually develop into melanoma. Also called a *dysplastic nevus.*

Basal cell carcinoma (BCC)—The most common form of skin cancer. BCC arises in the lower, or basal, layer of the epithelium. It rarely spreads beyond the skin but may be locally aggressive and invasive if not treated.

Benign—Not malignant or cancerous. A benign lesion lacks the ability to invade nearby tissues, blood vessels, or lymphatic channels.

Biopsy—Surgical removal of a lesion or part of a lesion so that it can be examined under a microscope to make a diagnosis.

Blue nevus—Dark blue/black mole usually rounded, firm, and sharply demarcated. Found often on the head and scalp. These nevi only rarely develop into melanoma (malignant blue nevus).

Breslow's depth—Measurement in millimeters of the depth of invasion of a primary melanoma from the dermal-epidermal junction to the most deeply invading melanoma cells. Breslow's depth is one of two major methods by which the depth of invasion of a primary melanoma is determined; the other method is the use of Clark's levels.

Carcinogens—Chemicals or other toxic agents, such as cigarette smoke or ultraviolet radiation, that are able to damage DNA and thereby increase the risk of cancer.

Cell division—The process by which a cell makes an exact copy, or clone, of itself. This process is normally very carefully regulated to prevent the production of too many or too few of a given type of cell.

Chemotherapy—Technically, a term referring to the use of drugs to treat disease, but usually used to refer to the use of chemical agents (drugs) to treat cancer.

Clark's levels—One of two major methods used to measure the depth of invasion of a primary melanoma. This method—developed by Dr. Wallace Clark, a physician who did a lot of important work in melanoma—is based on the deepest layer of skin the melanoma cells penetrate. The other method is Breslow's depth.

Clear margins—The presence of normal skin surrounding every border of a surgically removed malignant lesion. Clear margins suggest that all cancer cells have been removed locally. The presence of clear margins, however, does not assure that cancer cells have not invaded into blood vessels or lymphatic channels prior to removal of the lesion. See also **Positive margins.**

Clinical—A generic medical term, often used to refer to how a disease such as melanoma appears to the physician on physical examination, as opposed to pathologic examination under the microscope.

Clinical stage—The stage assigned to a tumor based on the original biopsy (which made the diagnosis of cancer) and clinical parameters only, such as the physical examination, blood tests, and scans. See also **Staging** and **Pathologic stage.**

Clone—Literally means "an exact duplicate of." In cancer, multiple different clones are generated when cancer cells proliferate, because mutations occur randomly during the dividing process.

Common acquired nevi—See **Acquired nevi.**

Complete remission (CR)—The apparent disappearance, after treatment, of all cancer cells detectable by blood tests, scanning techniques, or physical examination. This does not necessarily mean cure, since deposits of cancer that are too small to be detected by modern means may still be present and cause problems later.

Compound nevus—A mole whose melanocytes (nevus cells) are present both at the dermal-epidermal junction and in the dermal layers of the skin.

Congenital nevus—A mole that is present from birth, as opposed to an acquired nevus, which arises after birth. Congenital nevi are present in 1 out of 100 people of all races. They vary in size from a few millimeters to very large (see **Giant congenital nevus**).

Control—An individual or a group in an experimental study that does not receive the experimental treatment or procedure. The control group provides the standard against which the experimental treatment is judged.

Controlled trial—A research study that includes a group of patients who do not receive the experimental treatment but, rather, receive either the best proven treatment available at the time the study begins, no treatment, or a placebo. This "control group" provides a comparison with the experimental group so that researchers can determine whether or not the new treatment is better, worse, or equivalent to no treatment or the best current treatment. See also **Uncontrolled trial.**

CT or CAT (computerized axial tomography) scan—A means of viewing the organs and structures inside the body through the use of X rays and computer-generated pictures on film.

Cutaneous—Derived from, or relating, to the skin.

Cytokines—Specialized proteins produced by cells to send chemical messages to neighboring cells, particularly the cells of the immune system. Examples include the interferons and the interleukins.

De novo—Literally meaning "arising anew." A de novo melanoma is one that arises not from an existing mole but, rather, directly from a single melanocyte located at the dermal-epidermal junction.

Dermal-epidermal junction—The border between the outer two layers of skin where melanocytes normally reside.

Dermis—The second, or middle, layer of skin.

Dissection—See **Resection.**

DNA (deoxynucleic acid)—The "brain" or information-containing material present in the nucleus of every cell. DNA is made up of thousands of different genes. The genetic material contained within a cell's DNA controls the cell's ability to divide (make another copy, or clone, of itself), and orchestrates all of the cell's activities.

DTIC (Dacarbazine)—The chemotherapy drug most commonly used to treat metastatic melanoma.

Dysplastic nevus syndrome—See **Atypical mole syndrome.**

Dysplastic nevus—See **Atypical mole.**

Elective regional lymph node dissection—See **Lymph node dissection.**

Epidermis—The outermost layer of skin, composed of keratinocytes, the cells of origin of non-melanoma skin cancer.

Epiluminescence microscopy—A new method of examining pigmented lesions using a very bright light and magnification. It is hoped that this technique will allow doctors to determine which moles are likely to become precancerous or cancerous without removing them.

Familial atypical mole and melanoma syndrome (FAMM)—See **Atypical mole syndrome.**

Fine needle aspiration (FNA)—A commonly used, simple office procedure done to determine whether a swollen lymph gland or lump (say, in the breast or the thyroid gland) contains cancer. A needle is inserted into the lump or lymph node, and cells are sucked into an attached syringe and then examined microscopically for evidence of cancer. See Chapter 8.

First-degree relatives—A patient's parents, children, and siblings.

Follow-up—Return visits to a doctor or clinic for the purpose of determining the status of a medical problem.

Fotemustine—A relatively new chemotherapy drug that has been reported to have some success in treating advanced melanoma, including brain metastases.

Gallium scan—A type of imaging study that uses an injection of the radioisotope gallium to identify metastases. In theory, the cancer cells should take up the gallium, while normal cells should not. A nuclear medicine scan is used following the gallium injection to "light up" the areas of the body that have taken up the gallium.

Gamma knife—See **Stereotactic radiosurgery.**

Gene therapy—Treatments that use the injection or inhalation of DNA in attempt to treat a disease. Most types of gene therapy are still in the experimental stages.

Genes—Stretches of DNA, each of which codes for a molecule or protein with a highly specific function. For example, there is a particular gene contained within each cell's DNA that codes for insulin and another that codes for interferon. Every molecule or protein in the body is encoded for by its own gene.

Germline mutation—A gene that is inherited in a damaged form and passed on in that form from generation to generation in families. Because the damage is inherited, it is present in every cell in the body. This is in contrast to an acquired mutation, which occurs some time after birth and is then present only in a single set of cells such as a cancer.

Giant congenital nevus—A large mole present at the time of birth, most commonly found on the back, buttocks, chest, and shoulders. Giant congenital nevi are dark brown or black with a hairy, pebbly surface. They may extend deep under the skin into muscle and may even involve the covering of the spinal cord (leptomeninges). Five to ten percent develop melanoma.

Halo nevus—A mole surrounded by a ring (halo) of skin that is white because it lacks pigment. The cause and significance of halo nevi is not known, but the belief is that, for some reason, the immune system attacked and destroyed the melanocytes surrounding the mole.

Hospice—A facility or service that provides palliative and supportive care for terminally ill persons and their families either directly (in-patient hospice) or on a consulting basis (home hospice).

Hutchinson's melanotic freckle—Another name for *lentigo maligna*.

Immunocompromised (also **immunosuppressed**)—Used to describe a defective immune system in, for example, people receiving powerful drugs to prevent organ rejection after a transplant or to treat an illness and those infected with the AIDS virus.

Immunotherapy—A general term used to describe treatments that use the immune system to help fight or prevent disease.

In transit metastases—Melanoma metastases that occur between the primary site of origin on the skin and the lymph nodes draining that area.

Inflammation—The body's response to irritation, injury, or infection. We see this response on the skin as redness, swelling, warmth, and pain. This reaction may also occur in the lymph nodes, causing pain and swelling.

Interleukin 2 (IL-2)—A cytokine protein produced in the body by T lymphocytes in response to an antigenic (foreign) stimulus. It, in turn, stimulates the proliferation of other cells of the immune system. IL-2 has been manufactured and is used to treat some human cancers, including melanoma.

Intradermal nevus—A mole whose melanocytes (nevus cells) are present only in the dermis.

Intraoperative lymphatic mapping—A relatively new technique used in conjuction with lymphoscintigraphy and sentinel node biopsy to determine which lymph nodes are draining the site of the primary melanoma. This is used only for patients with a positive sentinel node biopsy to allow the surgeon to remove all other lymph nodes that may also contain melanoma.

Invasive—Used to describe a cancer cell that has spread to parts of the body that its normal or noncancerous counterpart cell is not able to spread to. In melanoma, *invasive* specifically refers to cancerous melanocytes (or melanoma cells) that have penetrated from the skin's dermal-epidermal junction, where they normally reside, down into the dermis, where they may then invade blood vessels or lymphatic channels, allowing spread to the internal organs. The ability of a cell to invade is the primary distinction between a cancer cell and a normal cell.

Junctional nevus—A mole in which the melanocytes (or nevus cells) are confined to the junction between the epidermis and dermis of the skin

Keratinocytes—Cells that make up the outer layer of skin (the epidermis). These are the cells from which nonmelanoma skin cancer originates.

Lentigo—The medical term for "old age spot" or "liver spot." Lentigos appear as flat brown spots, most commonly on the hands and face, of middle-aged and elderly people. They may gradually develop into a precancerous form called a lentigo maligna, which in turn may develop into a subtype of melanoma called lentigo maligna melanoma.

Lentigo maligna—A precancerous lentigo. A lentigo maligna is to a lentigo as an atypical (or dysplastic) mole is to a mole. Also sometimes called *Hutchinson's melanotic freckle.*

Lentigo maligna melanoma—A type of melanoma that develops from a lentigo rather than from a mole but is similar in every other way to melanoma arising from a mole.

Leptomeninges—The membranes covering the brain and spinal cord. These membranes may contain melanocytes, and on very rare occasions, melanoma may develop in them.

Lesion—The generic and commonly used medical term for any growth— benign or malignant—on the skin or other body organ.

Lymph nodes—Specialized swellings in the lymphatic vessels where infection-fighting immune cells collect. There are lymph nodes in many areas of the body, including the neck, armpits, groin, and many internal sites. These may become temporarily swollen and sore when the body is fighting an infection. Less commonly, they may become swollen when cancer cells spread there.

Lymph node dissection—The surgical removal of a group of lymph nodes for prognostic and/or treatment purposes in a patient known to have cancer. The removed lymph nodes are examined under a microscope to see if they contain cancer cells. *Regional lymph node dissection* refers to the removal of lymph nodes in the region believed to drain the site of origin of the primary tumor. *Elective regional lymph node dissection* means that the procedure is done, not out of medical necessity (as is often required when lymph nodes become so enlarged that they compress local nerves or blood vessels), but rather, in hopes of improving patient outcome.

Lymphatic channels—A network of small tubes or vessels that carry the lymph fluid throughout the body. This fluid contains lymphocytes and other cells of the immune system. The lymphatic channels are connected to the lymph nodes and the infection-fighting organs (bone marrow, spleen, and thymus).

Lymphoscintigraphy—A scan that uses a special radioactive tracer to determine which lymph node area or areas drain the site on the skin where a melanoma arose. The radioactive tracer is injected into the skin at the site of the primary melanoma, and different lymph node areas are then scanned. Any lymph nodes draining the site will light up on the scan.

Malignant—Another term for *cancerous*, or having the ability to invade nearby tissues, blood vessels, or lymphatic channels, allowing spread of the cancer cells to other parts of the body.

Melanin—The pigment produced by melanocytes that gives skin its color and allows tanning to occur. Melanin provides protection for keratinocytes and melanocytes against ultraviolet light, since UV light may damage their DNA. Naturally dark-skinned people produce both a darker form of melanin and a larger amount of melanin than do fair-skinned people.

Melanocytes—Cells that produce the protective pigment melanin. Melanocytes normally reside at the dermal-epidermal junction of skin, but they are also present in other areas of the body, including the retina of the eye and the linings of the mouth, anus, rectum, vagina, and spinal cord. Lentigos, moles, and melanoma all develop from melanocytes.

Melanoma—A cancer arising from melanocytes; also referred to as *malignant melanoma.*

Melanoma in situ—Melanoma in which the malignant cells have spread sideways along the dermal-epidermal junction but have not yet spread downwards to invade the dermis. Removal of a melanoma in situ lesion should result in cure because there are no blood vessels or lymphatics present at or above the dermal-epidermal junction. Other terms for *melanoma in situ* are *noninvasive melanoma* and *Clark's level I melanoma.*

Metastasis—A mass of cancer cells distant from the initial tumor site. Metastases develop when cells of the original tumor invade blood vessels or lymphatics and find a new site where they can proliferate.

Micrometastasis—A small collection of cancer cells that has spread from the site of origin of the initial tumor but has not formed a large enough tumor to be detected by the naked eye, blood tests, or imaging tests. Micrometastases are usually so small that they do not cause symptoms or problems, but unfortunately, they may later grow into larger tumors that do.

Microscopy—See **Epiluminescence microscopy.**

Mole—A cluster of melanocytes—all clones of a single melanocyte—that appears as a brown spot on the skin. The medical term for a mole is a *nevus.* Most melanomas are thought to arise from moles.

Monoclonal antibodies—See **Antibodies.**

MRI (magnetic resonance imaging)—A technique that uses powerful magnets to obtain X ray-like images (scans) of the inside of the body. In the case of melanoma, MRI scans are most often used to evaluate for brain metastases.

Mutation—A change in the genetic material (DNA) of a cell that may eventually result in the development of cancer. Mutations may arise from exposure to carcinogens, or they may arise spontaneously because of errors in cell division.

Nevus; plural **nevi**—The medical term for *mole.*

Nevus cells—Specialized melanocytes that make up moles.

Nucleus—The "brain" of the cell. DNA is stored in the nucleus of the cell.

Ocular—Pertaining to the eye.

Ocular melanoma—Melanoma arising in the eye.

Oncogene—A cancer-causing gene, usually arising from a mutated normal gene called a proto-oncogene. Just as there are many different proto-oncogenes, there are many different oncogenes.

Oncologist—A physician who specializes in the study and treatment of cancer.

Oncology—The medical field dedicated to the study and treatment of cancer.

Ophthalmologist—A medical doctor specializing in disorders of the eye.

Overall response rate—The total percentage of patients acheiving either a complete response or a partial response to a particular treatment. For example, if the complete response rate is 10% and the partial response rate is 25%, then the overall response rate is 35%.

p16—One of the tumor suppressor genes responsible for regulating or holding in check the growth of melanocytes. The p16 gene is often missing or damaged in melanoma cells, contributing to uncontrolled growth.

Partial remission (PR)—A decrease in size of all detectable cancer metastases by 50% or more in response to treatment.

Pathologic stage—The most accurate stage, based on the results of pathologic examination of tissue samples (biopsies). For example, if a Clark's level V melanoma is removed from a patient's leg and a physical examination, blood tests, and scans do not show any evidence of melanoma elsewhere, that patient's clinical stage would be stage II. However, if a patient undergoes a lymph node dissection and the pathologist finds melanoma in one or more of the lymph nodes, then the patient would be a (pathologic) stage III. See also **Staging** and **Clinical stage.**

Pathologist—A physician who specializes in the diagnosis of disease based on the microscopic appearance of body tissues.

PET (positron emission tomography) scan—A nuclear medicine scan used to detect metastases using a radioactive form of glucose that is administered intravenously and then taken up by cancer cells, where it gives off a radioactive signal that can be detected through use of a body-scanning machine.

Placebo—Any dummy medical treatment. "A sugar pill." Used in controlled clinical research trials to determine if the effects of the experimental treatment are real and specific. Usually, half of the people in the study are given the placebo, and half are given the treatment under study. The clinical outcomes of the two groups are then compared.

Positive margins—The presence of malignant cells extending to the border of a surgically removed specimen. Positive margins are highly suggestive that some cancer cells were left behind in the area where the surgery took place. The presence of positive margins is therefore an absolute indication for an additional resection to obtain clear margins.

Premalignant—Literally meaning "precancerous," *premalignant* refers to cellular changes that are not severe enough to allow the process of invasion (which defines the malignant state) to occur. If premalignant cells are left alone, further changes may occur, leading to outright cancer. Atypical moles are the premalignant form (or precursor) to melanoma, just as colon polyps are the premalignant form of colon cancer.

Primary—A term frequently used to refer to the initial melanoma arising on the skin, as in the phrase "the primary lesion" or just "the primary." The primary is in contrast to melanoma that has traveled, or metastasized, to a distant site. Melanoma that has spread away from the primary lesion is called a *metastasis,* a *recurrence,* or *recurrent* or *metastatic disease.* A new cancerous mole is a new primary, not a recurrence of another primary.

Prognosis—The expected outlook for a patient with a disease, based on statistics generated from other patients with the same disease.

Prognostic factors—Clinical and laboratory variables (e.g., gender, age, or depth of invasion of the primary tumor) that have been determined by research studies to be linked to either a good or a bad outcome. There are both good and bad prognostic factors.

Proliferation—The process of repeated cell divisions.

Protein—Molecules made by the body and essential for its functioning, such as insulin and antibodies. Each protein is encoded for by its own gene.

Proto-oncogene—A normal gene involved in controlling cell division. There are many different proto-oncogenes.

Punch biopsy—The most commonly used technique to remove a skin lesion for microscopic analysis. A small, round cookie-cutter-like tool, which comes in various sizes ranging from 2 to 10 millimeters, is used to remove the lesion and a small amount of skin around and under it. Depending on the size of the punch used, one or a few stiches may be needed to close the small wound.

Recurrence—The emergence of melanoma at a site distant from the primary lesion (metastasis), often many months or years after the initial diagnosis.

Regional lymph node dissection—See **Lymph node dissection.**

Relative risk—A numerical estimate of the influence of a particular characteristic, such as hair color, on the likelihood of developing a particular disease. The number compares the risk of a person with the characteristic with the risk of the population as a whole. For example, if you have blond or red hair, you have a melanoma risk factor of 2 to 3. This means you are twice to three times as likely as the "average" person to develop melanoma. A relative risk of less than 1 would imply that the characteristic gives you a less-than-average chance of developing the disease. People with few or no moles have a risk factor of 0.3. This means they are only a third as likely as the average person to develop the disease.

Remission—The disappearance of a disease, but not necessarily a cure. In cancer treatment the terms *complete remission* (complete disappearance of all evidence of the cancer) and *partial remission* (a decrease in size by 50% or more of all known areas of cancer) are used.

Resection—Medical term for the surgical removal of tissue or organs. In reference to lymph node removal, the term *dissection* is commonly used and is, in this case, synonymous with *resection.*

Risk factors—Personal characteristics or habits such as age, gender, skin color, or cigarette smoking that have been found in research studies to be associated with a higher-than-average likelihood of developing a particular disease.

Seborrheic keratosis—A benign pigmented lesion with a characteristic raised, dark, waxy, "stuck-on" appearance. Seborrheic keratoses occur with increasing frequency with advancing age, but they are not at risk of becoming melanoma.

Sentinel lymph node biopsy—Surgical removal (biopsy) of the lymph node identified by lymphoscintigraphy to be the first lymph node to drain the area of the primary melanoma. The surgical specimen is then examined under a microscope for the presence of melanoma cells. If melanoma cells are found, a lymph node dissection will usually then be performed.

Sentinel lymph node—The first lymph node to drain the area on the skin where there is a melanoma or where one has been removed. Its location is determined by lymphoscintigraphy.

SPF (solar protective factor)—The number present on all sunscreens which rates the degree of sun protection they provide. An SPF of 6 means that one can stay in the sun on average six times longer than is possible without sunscreen and still avoid sunburn. (Remember, however, that the sun can still damage the skin and increase the risk of melanoma even if one does not get a sunburn.)

Spitz nevus—A type of benign mole most often arising in children and young adults that may be confused with melanoma because it looks similar to melanoma under the microscope. Also called *benign juvenile melanoma* (a contradiction in terms).

Squamous cell carcinoma (SCC)—Cancer of the epithelial cells usually arising in sun-damaged skin. Initially local and superficial, these cancers may invade and metastasize if unattended.

Staging—A series of studies, including physical examinations, X rays, blood tests, and sometimes surgery, aimed at identifying if and where a tumor has spread beyond the region in which it initially arose. For most types of cancer, research studies have provided an estimation of the prognosis associated with each tumor stage.

Statistically significant—A commonly used term in medical research meaning that a study's conclusion has been shown by rigid statistical analysis to be—with at least a 95% certainty—due to the intervention under study (and not to chance alone). Only statistically significant findings are accepted by the medical community.

Stereotactic radiosurgery—A specialized technique allowing the delivery of radiation beams to a very precise area shown to contain tumor cells so that the number of normal cells exposed to the radiation may be reduced. In melanoma, it is most often used for brain metastases. A similar technique using somewhat different machinery is known as the *Gamma knife.*

Subcutaneous fat—The third and deepest layer of skin, composed of fat, blood vessels, and lymphatic channels.

Subcutaneous nodules—Lumps under the skin. In melanoma often a sign of local recurrence at or near the site where a primary melanoma has been removed.

Subungual melanoma—Melanoma arising under the fingernails or toe-nails.

Temazolamide—A new drug used in chemotherapy for advanced melanoma. It is similar to DTIC but can be given by mouth.

Tumor suppressor genes—Genes that play an important role in regulating the proliferation of normal cells. If more than one of these genes is damaged or lost, the loss of control may result in cancer. Tumor suppressor genes do not suppress tumors that are already present, as their name implies.

Tyrosinase—A protein involved in the production of melanin that is made only by melanocytes and melanoma cells. A blood test for tyrosinase is currently being studied to determine whether it will allow detection of melanoma metastases that are too small to be detected by other means.

Ultraviolet (or UV) radiation—A form of energy given off naturally by the sun or artificially by tanning booth lights that is capable of burning the skin. It is also capable of damaging the DNA inside skin cells. This damage may, in turn, cause a previously normal cell to develop into a cancerous one. There are two types of UV radiation that reach the earth's surface, UVA and UVB. UVB is more likely to burn the skin and is thought to be associated with the development of both melanoma and nonmelanoma skin cancer. UVA is less likely to cause a sunburn because it penetrates more deeply into the skin, but it almost certainly does contribute to DNA damage. Thus, it is best to protect one's skin from both UVA and UVB.

Uncontrolled trial—A study that does not have a "control" group (one that receives a placebo or the best available treatment) to which the results of the treatment group may be compared. This type of study often produces misleading results and is most often used with small numbers of patients to see whether further study in a larger, controlled trial seems warranted. See also **Controlled trial.**

Vaccine—A suspension of material (proteins or cells) administered, usually by injection, with the goal of stimulating an immune response.

Vitiligo—A benign skin condition in which one or more patches of skin become white, due to the immune system's attack on melanocytes. Vitiligo is not related to the development of melanoma, and its cause is unknown.

Whole body photography—A technique used by pigmented lesion specialists to help keep track of changes in nevi in persons with the atypical mole syndrome. A series of photographs are taken which cover the body's entire skin surface. Close-up shots are also taken of moles with atypical features. Two sets of the photographs are made—one for the patient and one for the physician—to aid in earlier detection of changes in moles over time than may be possible otherwise.

Wide local excision—The surgical removal of a margin of normal skin around a site shown by a previous skin biopsy to contain melanoma. This is done to ensure that all the cancer cells in the area have been removed.

Index

Jill R. Schofield, M.D., is a graduate of the University of Colorado Medical School and did her residency training in internal medicine at the Johns Hopkins Hospital. She has had a long-standing interest in the development, prevention, and early detection of malignant melanoma, and in patient education. She currently works as an internist/hospitalist at St. Joseph Hospital for the Colorado Permanente Medical Group in Denver, Colorado.

William A. Robinson, M.D., Ph.D., is a graduate of the University of Colorado Medical School. He did his residency training in internal medicine at the Massachusetts General Hospital followed by oncology training and a Ph.D. at the Walter and Eliza Hall Institute, University of Melbourne, Australia. He directed the Melanoma Research Clinic at the University of Colorado for many years and has written extensively on the biology and treatment of melanoma. From 1996 to 1999 he was a visiting scientist at the Ludwig Institute for Cancer Research in Melbourne, further defining the genes and genetics of melanoma. He is currently the American Cancer Society Professor of Clinical Oncology at the University of Colorado Health Sciences Center in Denver.

Library of Congress Cataloging-in-Publication Data

Schofield, Jill R.
   What you really need to know about moles and melanoma / Jill R.
Schofield and William A. Robinson.
         p.   cm. —(A Johns Hopkins Press health book)
Includes index.
      ISBN 0-8018-6393-7 (hardcover : acid-free paper) — ISBN 0-8018-6394-5
(pbk. : acid-free paper)
      1. Melanoma—Popular works.   2. Mole (Dermatology)—Popular works.
I. Robinson, William A. 1934–   II. Title.   III. Series.
      RC280.M37 S36 2000
      616.99′477—dc21   00-008003